The Infertility Cleanse

Detox, Diet and Dharma
for Fertility

The Infertility Cleanse

Detox, Diet and Dharma for Fertility

Tami Quinn, Beth Heller

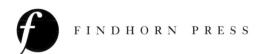 FINDHORN PRESS

First published by Findhorn Press 2011

ISBN: 978-1-84409-508-7

British Library Cataloguing-in-Publication Data.
A catalogue record for this book is available from the British Library.

Cover and Interior designed by Damian Keenan
Printed and bound in China

1 2 3 4 5 6 7 8 9 10 20 19 18 17 16 15 14 13 12 11

Published by
Findhorn Press
117-121 High Street,
Forres IV36 1AB Scotland,
United Kingdom

t +44-(0)1309-690582
f +44(0)131-777-2711
e info@findhornpress.com
www.findhornpress.com

Table of Contents

Dedications

We wrote this book during one of the most challenging years we can ever remember. In addition to a crashing economy and trying to find balance between work and family, our offices at Pulling Down the Moon were completely flooded by the Chicago River and destroyed in July of 2010. Since then, we've rebuilt our space, written this book and somehow ended up stronger than ever. During these times of what we call "flood and famine," we were supported by many people who helped us survive and thrive. The field of Integrative Care for Fertility is rapidly evolving, primarily from the insight of those thick in the work. The commitment of our practitioners and the stories and the experiences of our patients guide us in all we do at Pulling Down the Moon. Our heartfelt thanks go out to the following:

Matt Heller, Brian Quinn, Kriyananda, the practitioners at Pulling Down the Moon, Thierry Bogliolo, Nicky Leach, Ali Domar, Marie Davidson, Caitlin Roche, the physicians at Fertility Centers of Illinois and Shady Grove Fertility, Mimi Productions.

We are also extremely grateful for our ever evolving yoga practice and its persistent, subtle presence in our lives and work.

Most importantly, we dedicate The Infertility Cleanse to our children: Kevin, Courtney, Jackson and Calvin. May they see through this book that despite hardships in life, the strength to blossom and grow is always there when we follow our heart and its good intentions.

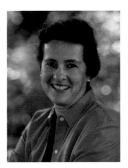

Foreword

I met Tami Quinn and Beth Heller about ten years ago, when they asked me to speak at the opening of Pulling Down the Moon, their first integrative care center for infertility. Since then, our paths have crossed with increasing frequency, to the point now where we are actually talking about partnering in the creation of a new model of integrative care centers.

Our relationship has been challenged from time to time, however, by my obsession with maintaining strict scientific standards. Tami and Beth are visionaries, yoga teachers, and caregivers. I am the nerd. They speak of caring for the souls of their patients. I talk about statistical significance and randomized controlled studies. They use the word "can." I use the word "may."

So you can imagine my horror when they told me the title of their new book. The Infertility Cleanse as a title gave me visions of coffee enemas, ultra-elimination diets, and toxic herbs. I could not believe that at least some of my scientific rigor had not rubbed off on them. So I told them of my extreme concern and they reassured me that the book was indeed based on science, that I needed to trust them, offered to let me read the galleys, and invited me to write the foreword if in fact I was comfortable with the content.

Since you are currently reading a foreword by me, you can guess that I did read the book, and am comfortable with the content. But the scientist in me (ok, nerd) had to come to terms with the word "cleanse." So of course I looked it up in the thesaurus.

Cleanse means to absolve, clarify, clean, clear, depurgate, disinfect, expurgate, launder, lustrate, purge, purify, refine, restore, sanitize, scour, scrub, or sterilize. I have actually never seen or used the words depurgate or expurgate, but in terms of infertility treatment from a holistic point of view, I like the concepts of restoration, clarification, and refinement. But a book called "Infertility Refinement" just doesn't do it. So I had to come to terms with the word "cleanse."

There are a lot of unknowns in the field of infertility treatment. Although the vast majority of individuals and couples who see an infertility specialist get a definitive diagnosis, not everyone who is treated conceives and delivers a baby. And in fact, most of the normal appearing embryos transferred as part of an IVF cycle don't implant. So, there is room in this equation for other factors to play a role: factors such as diet, stress, and the environment. I have spent most of my research career focusing on the relationship between stress and fertility and I believe that we now have data to support the fact that stress is a detriment to conception, and that teaching women specific stress reduction strategies is associated with significant increases in pregnancy rates. Although we don't have the gold standard, randomized controlled trials, to prove that the other interventions covered in this book increase pregnancy rates, we do know that these strategies have helped other patient populations, there aren't any downsides to improving your diet and adopting healthier lifestyle habits, and anything one can do to increase one's sense of control leads to peace of mind. And trust me, if you have peace of mind, you have everything.

Alice D. Domar, Ph.D.

Photo courtesy of Barbara Peacock Photography

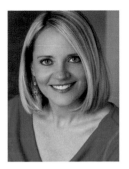

Tami's Cleansing Moment

"Now bend your knee and sink into Warrior 2." The yoga teacher's instructions were clear, yet I somehow couldn't hear exactly what she was saying through the static clouding my brain. My body was in the yoga room, but my mind was simultaneously in a million places. It was a day I was supposed to be "working from home," but I chose to break the stress of my day with a yoga class just around the corner.

I was new to this practice of yoga; it wasn't considered particularly "hip," and God only knew if it could help me shed the 10 pounds I was never able to lose after the twins were born. Nonetheless, I knew I had to try something to pull me out of the three-year slump I was in—the slump that made me cry all the time, feel moody, completely burned-out, tender, stressed, and alone. I was so blessed in so many ways, yet nothing seemed to make sense anymore. I had struggled so hard to have my twins, and now that I had them, why was I leaving them with a nanny four days a week so I could go to a job that stressed me out beyond belief? I wasn't feeling very healthy lately, either. Constant headaches, numbness and tingling in my arms and legs, chronic sinus infections. The neurologist did an MRI hoping to eliminate the possibility of MS. The results came back negative, and he asked me if I felt stressed a lot. "Hell yeah," I said, "You got a test for that?"

"Now, breathe deeply and see if you can go a little further in the pose."

I was back in the yoga room again, but then came my next static-filled visual. Pound, pound, pound. "Mommy, are you in there? Open the door and stop working on your computer. We want you to come with Tonia and us to the park."

"I can't right now, honey, maybe a little later." Sigh, then those familiar tears streaming down my face again. Stop it. Push through. Back to work. The devil on my shoulder suddenly appeared and was making a compelling argument."Remember how it goes? Work now, play later! You can't be fully present with them anyway. Not when you're thinking about your 'to do' list back here in the home office."

I had attempted every permutation of flex-time imaginable, and my employer tried to accommodate me any way they could. I tried working from home one day per week, part-time, even job sharing, but ultimately ended up making less money for the same amount of work. Nothing seemed workable. Giving up the job didn't make sense either. I made too much money. How could we afford to lose half of our income? Could we pay the mortgage? What about my career? I'd worked so hard to be successful at Martha Stewart Living, but those twins... my god, how can I leave them everyday? Every fiber of my being just wants to be with them.

I was back in the yoga room again. Thankfully, we were on the floor doing cobra pose. This would allow me a chance to check if I had any missed calls on my cell phone. I had set it next to my mat and put it on "silent," but at least I could see if anybody at the office was trying to reach me. Damn, a missed call from New York, probably my publisher at the magazine.

We pushed back into downward facing dog, I picked up my cell phone, walked outside and called the New York number listed.

"Hey, Albert, it's Tami. Did you guys call?"

"Yeah, Sylvia's looking for you. She's on the warpath again today. Isn't hitting the ad sale numbers she promised Martha for the next issue. Hold on a minute, I'll put her on the phone."

"Where are you? I need a list of everybody you have lined up for the next issue. Call Target. See if they'll upgrade to a spread if we position them on cover 2, page 1. I need you to bring in at least two more pages by tomorrow. I don't want to hear about budget cuts and advertisers' marketing seasonality, just find the goddamn pages. Staff conference call in two hours. Be on it." Click.

"Inhale, take your arms up overhead, grab your wrist, hinge at the waist and exhale into half-moon."

I'm back inside and on my yoga mat again. I promised the kids I'd take them to the kids' museum later on today. They'll be heartbroken that we can't go. Maybe I can take the conference call on my cell while at the museum. I wonder if they have private rooms at that place. I look back down at the phone on my mat again. Did I just see another call come through? Is it the nanny or the kids? I'll have to leave class again and go outside. Phew, I imagined it. No calls. Wonder when this yoga practice is going to end. I need to get back on the phone.

I walked out of yoga class that day in a surreal state of being. My body felt open and relaxed from yoga, my mind felt completely agitated by my phone call, and my spirit felt broken and defeated. I went home, dropped to my knee, and cried like a baby.

Suddenly, I felt out of body. I noticed there was something watching me cry, it was me but a me I didn't recognize. This me just sort of watched detachedly, and then said, "If you're so miserable, change it. You keep waiting for answers or some big event that will prompt change in your life, but you are the change you seek. It's not an event outside you; it's within you. What are you waiting for?"

It was like some divine Awareness that cut through the crap of everything going on in that moment. An Awareness that knew me and my story and was empowering me to take ownership of my life and write the story the way I wanted it to be written. I wouldn't call it an "Aha moment,"—more like a period of awakening.

Through the next several weeks I began to sit with the idea of letting go. Letting go of the career I had painted in my mind, letting go of the money I thought I needed, letting go of the ego, which proudly boasted of my enviable position in advertising. Most importantly, letting go of the story I thought I could have of being the mother of twins, a wife, homemaker, a highly successful advertising executive and a happy, healthy, whole person. I looked at my phone. It became a symbol of everything that was wrong with my life. I was waiting for the call that would give me answers, but it never came.

I started going to more yoga classes. I left my cell phone at home. One day my teacher mentioned this place called The Temple of Kriya Yoga. I read online about the in-depth classes they offered in yoga and spirituality. I felt inspired by this man they called Kriyananda. He spoke of things I had never heard before, yet somehow they struck a note inside of me and felt oddly familiar. I read yoga books, started meditating again, bought tapes of Kriyananda's lectures, went to more yoga classes, changed my diet, started using a neti pot and learned to tune out my cell phone. I was detoxifying and starting to feel healthy again. I knew what I had to do.

I let go of my job in advertising and everything it symbolized. I became a yoga teacher and asked Kriyananda to be my spiritual guru. We cut back and lived more simply, but I felt happier. Somehow the bills got paid and I spent glorious days with my twins at the park, at the children's museum, or baking cookies at home. Ironically, about nine months later, my husband started making more money. Today, he has far surpassed the deficit created when I stopped working. I met Beth. Together we created Pulling Down the Moon, a new career, and my life's work based on the principles of yoga. My cleanse had worked. One part of me died, but something better had been born.

My twins are nearly 14, and as I write this, I find tears streaming down my cheeks once again. Where has the time gone? Did I miss those early years of their life when I never felt truly present? As Pulling Down the Moon sits on the brink of becoming a national company, am I fully present now as college lurks just four years away when they will leave this nest for good?

While pondering this question, an email pops into my inbox from one of my kids' teachers:

Dear Tami,

What a great article about you in The New York Times! You are a famous lady! And doing a great service to us ladies!

I wish I had you around 32 years ago when I was 33 and trying to get pregnant. I finally gave up because I was so stressed out and said "If God wants us to have children, then we will have them. I'm not doing all this stuff anymore!!"

The stress was gone, and I completely forgot about it, and three months later I was pregnant two months and didn't even remember missing a period. Stress is a killer!

I wish I had known you then!

Keep up the good work, lady!!!! I am very very proud of you!!

I finish reading the email and step into Awareness once again. I hear these words, "No regrets. Everything is exactly as it should be."

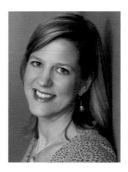

Beth's Cleansing Moment

*"You are not obligated, or even advised,
to believe your own thoughts."*

These words, which flew into my ears from my iPod, were incredibly simple; yet they set in motion of a chain of events in my life that has proved profound. When they made contact, I was driving my car and listening to a dharma talk by Gil Fronsdal. Over the last few months, listening to Gil's teachings while I drove was one way I was keeping it together.

To set the stage for why this simple phrase brought about such a "could have had a V-8" moment, let me tell you a bit about the last year. First of all, it goes almost without saying that if you've lived in the United States at any point since 2008 you can attest that this period has been one of the most troubling and toxic times since the Great Depression—especially for business owners. In July of 2010, in the midst of the general economic misery, the Chicago office of Pulling Down the Moon, which is located in a beautiful spot along the Chicago River, was destroyed by a fluke flood. As Tami and I watched the river waters recede we knew our regularly massive to-do list now included moving to a temporary space, caring for our patients during this transition, and continuing to grow as a business—all from a not-so-ideal temporary home. On a personal level, two weeks prior to the deluge, my oldest brother shared with the family that he'd been diagnosed with cancer. Two weeks following the flood my other brother, who is in many ways my soulmate, filed for divorce from his wife of 20 years and was struggling with how to explain this breakup to his beautiful son.

After these bruising months, I felt like I had a bullseye on my back. Each time a phone rang I wondered what trauma was waiting for me on the other end. The sense of dread became so bad that even the small beams of good news and success that broke through these heavy clouds made me feel dangerously exposed—as if any good fortune in the midst of all this suffering was somehow to be punished. I hadn't felt like this since… well, since I was struggling with infertility.

Ironically, I was simultaneously writing this book—a book that outlines a philosophy of living that can bolster the body and mind to withstand a toxic environment. It is designed to help women survive and thrive during their fertility struggles. Yet, from where I sat at my computer, life as I knew it had become frightening, sad, and, well, utterly toxic. I had firm faith in the techniques in use at Pulling Down the Moon—I had seen them help thousands of women and experienced the gifts of my own yoga practice—but here I was: a failure at my own game. How could I expound solutions when life was giving me the whipping of the century? And then that phrase.

"You are not obligated, or even advised, to believe your own thoughts."

As both a teacher and student of meditation, I am quite familiar with thoughts. For years I have observed what thoughts are, what thoughts aren't, how thoughts dance a manic dance, and how they are slippery and seldom based in reality. I use meditation daily, like "mental floss," to clear out confusion, untangle my emotional response to life situations, and to simply live more consciously. But in this overwhelming situation I started to feel as if I was meditating on a sinking ship. And the worst part was that I knew my thoughts were not grounded in reality. While a lot of bad stuff had gone down, I was still standing. Why in the midst of life, surrounded by a fantastic husband and the beautiful family I'd struggled so hard to create, was I not filled with gratitude that I was alive and well? Negative thoughts crashed over me like waves for literally months and I simply couldn't find a life raft. Until I heard that phrase.

"You are not obligated, or even advised, to believe your own thoughts."

I don't know why I heard that phase so clearly that day, but maybe my inner Awareness had had enough of Little Miss Misery. Those of you who read Fully Fertile may remember that my "a-ha" moment about my body, mind, and fertility came while I was running on a treadmill. Now the "a-ha" came when these simple words slammed into the treadmill of toxicity that was running in my mind. I was not these thoughts and not this misery. However, I was the energy that was allowing them to race on. Could it be so simple? Could I just pull the plug on the negative thought treadmill in my mind?

I get chills when I'm on to something.

That very night, I had a tremendous dream. I dreamed that my husband Matt and I had purchased a new home. The house was amazingly beautiful and made entirely of windows. Inside, it was decorated in rich colors and had an enormous fireplace that filled it with light and warmth.

 In the dream there was only joy and excitement—all fear, dread, and foreboding had evaporated. Upon waking, I wrote the dream down because I knew it was "a biggie." I had been given a glimpse into the truth of my own being. I had an opportunity, the dream seemed to say, to inhabit this beautiful place—nurture it and fill it with love. Interestingly, the house was made of glass. The windows seemed to be saying that it was futile to build walls to keep out pain. Perhaps the old adage "People who live in glass houses should not throw stones" was also at work. In the previous months, as I watched all the suffering around me I had fixated on my own vulnerability—the bullseye I imagined on my back, the stones that imagined enemies would hurl at me. These glass walls weren't fragile, though; they made me feel safe.

I woke from the dream feeling fresh and restored, with a new awareness of my center. The house's transparency seemed to be an invitation to look inside and shine the light of Awareness into my heart and mind. This dream confirmed that the advice I'd heard on the iPod was true. Negative thoughts—the waves of fear and stress—were not based in reality, and I didn't have to believe them.

The next day there were new questions. If I didn't have to believe my thoughts—if, in essence, my thoughts weren't based in reality—what was causing them? They had a persistence that showed they were drawing energy from somewhere. It was time to start looking deeper, to find and eliminate their source. Beyond these thoughts, what core belief needed to be brought into the light? Could I trust in this beautiful symbolic image of the glass house to begin to look inside for answers? The answer is yes. Symbols, as we have suggested, arise from patterns of thought and belief. My inner Awareness chose to send me the symbol of the house—a positive symbol of my core belief that I am whole and happy, which I had forgotten due to the "toxicity" of the last several months. If I chose to "move in" to this belief again, my dream symbol was telling me, I had a chance to create new, more positive patterns.

So move in I did. I sat in meditation and visualized my entire family moving in to this lovely house. I put a fire in the fireplace and a pot of soup on the stove. I resolved to become fearless—for nothing could shatter this place within me. These were not new or radical thoughts. As a yogi, the core belief in my own inner radiance is a guiding tenet; in the storm of negativity that was surrounding me, I had simply lost my way. From this point forward, life began to shift. The negative thoughts had less power and my inner radiance once again became my guiding light. The treadmill of negativity that was clouding my light, like the treadmill of stress that was impacting my fertility years ago, was no longer out of control. It had slowed and I was again in connection with a stronger Self. More than anything this experience drove home the recognition that a Cleanse Lifestyle is important for more than just fertility. It can change the rest of our lives. We hope it will change yours.

Disclaimer

BEFORE APPLYING any techniques described in this or any other nutrition, exercise, or holistic program, an individual should always consult and obtain professional medical advice, including from their doctor.

Not all of the techniques and exercises in this book may be suitable for all readers, and this and any other exercise program may result in physical injury. Women, whether pregnant or not, and men should consult their doctor before beginning any exercise, yoga or holistic program.

The patient-specific details, stories and narratives in this book have been altered to protect the patients' confidentiality. Names and identifying characteristics of the people have been changed. Specific references to websites, books or videos do not constitute an endorsement by the authors or publisher.

What is The Infertility Cleanse?

When we set out to write this book, we wanted to take a laywoman's stab at understanding the impact of toxic lifestyle factors on a woman's fertility and ability to conceive. The volume of interest about this topic from patients, the scientific community, and the media made us feel, as fertility specialists, that we needed to get to the bottom of this heated issue.

When we first presented the topic to our publisher—a book we naively chose to call *The Infertility Cleanse*—we were optimistic that we would be able to clearly define toxicity for the audience, and help women eradicate it to improve their fertility. But as so often happens, a topic that at first seems cut and dried in theory reveals its true nature the moment you sit down at your computer to actually write about it. And that was the case this time.

Toxicity, it seems, is everywhere. It's in our water bottles, the food we eat, and the air we breathe. Moreover, we are not simply passive inhabitants of a toxic wasteland; we are also active participants in the creation of mental, emotional, environmental, and physical toxicity through the ways we live our lives. In fact, the more we delved into the issue of toxicity, the more depressing the story became, and we began to look at each other and wonder how anyone ever gets pregnant or delivers a healthy child!

But as we dug deeper, the story changed and something else emerged. Nature has not left us defenseless in a toxic world. Somehow, despite all of the toxicity surrounding us, flowers are still blooming, trees are still growing, rain still falls, and families are still created. There is a resilience in nature that inspires us and gives us hope.

Rather than wallow in doom and gloom, we decided we would turn our energy to the ways our amazing bodies and spirits can overcome toxic challenges—a lifestyle cleanse, so to speak.

We reject the idea of toxicity as merely an external process—something from outside of ourselves trying to get in and cause harm. We believe toxicity is also something created internally that in turn manifests itself outwardly. Toxicity is a symbol of everything that's going wrong—patterns of stress, poor diet, inadequate sleep, and insufficient respect for the environment.

When we looked at toxicity this way, we had an epiphany: We each have a choice to change our lifestyle and choose another way to be. And that's what this book is all about.

Awareness and Proactivity

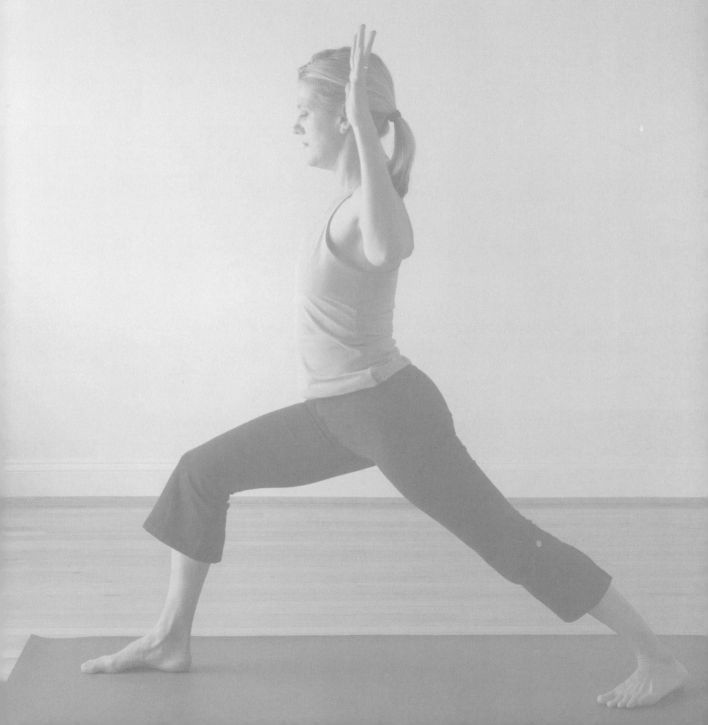

CHAPTER 1

The Body's Detox Processes

Each day our bodies are deluged with hundreds of things that could be called toxins. According to Webster's Dictionary, a toxin is defined as "a poisonous substance that is a specific product of the metabolic activities of a living organism." Toxins are a normal part of the natural world. Our bodies produce toxins, chemicals in our environment can be toxic to our bodies, and even mental health practitioners have co-opted the term to describe mental processes that can be harmful to our well-being. The important thing to realize is that toxicity is not something new to the human body.

For this reason, doom-and-gloom scenarios about the environment and our fertility must be taken seriously but also taken in stride. The keys to limiting the effects of toxins in our daily life are awareness and proactivity.

AWARENESS: THE MANY SOURCES OF TOXINS

While some toxins (i.e., poisonous chemicals) are dangerous in small amounts, most of the substances we talk about in this book are toxic only when the body's ability to metabolize and excrete these substances is overwhelmed or imbalanced. There are three main sources of toxins in our lives: environmental toxins, metabolic toxins, and xenobiotics.

1. Environmental Toxins

Environmental toxins come from the external environment. They are absorbed through the lungs (air pollution, smoking, fumes, cleaning products, certain artificial fragrances, etc.), through the food and drink we consume, and even through the use of some health and beauty products (perfumes, lotions, and skin care products). Toxins in the food supply enter the body through the digestive system and move directly to the liver, where they are cleared for excretion. Some examples of environmental toxins include:

HORMONES IN OUR FOOD SUPPLY: Our food supply is a significant source of chemicals, hormones, and hormone-like substances. In later sections of the book, we discuss the most significant sources of hormones and toxicity (animal products and pesticides) and strategies to reduce our consumption of these substances. Hormones in meat, dairy, and endocrine-disrupting pesticides (see below) can mimic the activity of our own endocrine hormones and disrupt normal function.

ENDOCRINE DISRUPTORS: Of particular concern for fertility is a family of exogenous toxins called endocrine disruptors. According to the National Institute of Environmental Health Sciences, endocrine disruptors are substances that interfere with our body's hormonal systems and cause adverse developmental, reproductive, neurological, and immune effects in humans and wildlife. They are associated with infertility and cancer, as well as developmental problems, and are found in many places, including pesticides, plastics, industrial byproducts, building materials, and pollution.

Unlike other toxins that must be ingested in large amounts before they cause problems, the hormones in the endocrine system that these chemicals mimic act in minute concentrations in our body. Many researchers believe that tiny amounts of endocrine disruptors have the potential to cause enormous damage. Common endocrine-disrupting chemicals include DDT, PCBs, Bisphenol A, and pthalates. These substances and their impact on health and fertility are discussed in greater depth later in the book.

2. Metabolic Toxins

Many of us don't realize that we may be our own biggest source of toxicity. The byproducts of normal cell metabolism and other physiological processes that originate in our body tissues are all toxic when they are not metabolized properly. Diet, overweight, stress, and a weakened digestive system can allow these substances to build up and begin to cause disease. Examples of toxins that result from our body's metabolic processes include excess hormones like insulin or estrogen and the byproducts of chronic inflammation and oxidative stress. These potential sources of toxicity are explored in the next chapter. Here are a few examples of metabolic processes that can become toxic:

ESTROGEN DOMINANCE: Too much estrogen circulating in a woman's body is thought to be a contributing factor toward infertility, endometriosis, and fibroids. During a woman's childbearing years, estrogen is made in two places: the ovaries and the adipose tissue (fat cells). Body fat is biologically active, and women who are overweight or obese may manufacture levels of estrogen in excess of healthy levels. In addition, the way a woman metabolizes estrogen is important to their health, too. Later we examine the different paths estrogen takes on the way out of the body and how these metabolic pathways can influence the amount and type of estrogen circulating in the body.

STRESS AND ITS METABOLITES: The stress hormone cortisol is a case of a good hormone gone wrong. Secreted by the adrenal glands, it evolved as part of our human response to danger and is called the "fight-or-flight" hormone. When out of control, stress can be one of the most toxic processes in our life.

INSULIN RESISTANCE: The metabolic hormone insulin is released by the pancreas in response to a meal and signals our cells to transport newly available blood sugar into the cells. When the body is chronically exposed to too many simple carbohydrates, insulin levels climb and cells lose their ability to respond to insulin's metabolic message. What results is a toxic, health-threatening condition called insulin resistance.

Insulin is essential for more than digestion and immediate energy needs. It sends excess glucose to the muscles and liver to be stored as glycogen for use later on (particularly overnight or during fasting); it signals excess sugar to be laid down as body fat; it stimulates the liver to produce cholesterol, which is key to the manufacture of healthy cell membranes and hormones; and its role in keeping blood sugar stable helps the body avoid chronic inflammation triggered by excess sugar, which can damage body tissues and lead to diabetes, heart disease, and other medical conditions. Most important, when it comes to fertility, insulin is chemically similar to the body's reproductive hormones. This can create confusion in the endocrine system that sets up disruption in the reproductive system and contributes to infertility in women with polycystic ovary syndrome (PCOS), or women who are overweight.

3. Xenobiotics

The term *xenobiotic* simply refers to "a chemical compound that is foreign to a living organism." Examples of xenobiotics include food additives that have been "proven safe" for human consumption and over-the-counter and pharmaceutical drugs, including fertility medications. The number of xenobiotics our bodies must cope with has increased with human medical and technological advancement. Xenobiotics are not necessarily bad for us (and in many cases may be beneficial, as with therapeutic herbs and medications); they are simply foreign to our physiology and must be managed by the body's detoxification systems. The more chemicals we encounter in our lives, the more complex this management project becomes. The key to managing xenobiotics is keeping our body's systems and defenses strong.

THE GOOD NEWS: PROACTIVITY

Okay, so that was the tough message. Now for the good news. We can take concrete steps to minimize our exposure to toxic substances, and there are effective strategies for enhancing the body's ability to manage environmental and internal stresses. In fact, the most amazing part of this story is the human body's flexibility in dealing with this onslaught of toxicity. While our genetic makeup hasn't changed much since cave-woman days, our environment has changed drastically.

Our bodies manage toxins in several ways. Mechanical systems that process toxins in the body include the lymphatic, circulatory, and integumentary systems, the latter involving perspiration/sloughing through the skin. The body's biochemical system involves the liver, the body's main detox organ, which is responsible for filtering out toxins in the blood and complex chemical reactions known as Phase 1 and Phase 2 known as biotransformation. We even host living creatures in our intestines ("good bacteria," or probiotics), which benefit the digestive system in many ways, including limiting our exposure to toxic substances. Finally, our mental processes play a vital role in detox. When we're supporting these body systems, our access to vibrant health is much improved.

Managing toxicity is a normal part of body function. In fact, the human body is constantly managing toxins. When our cells use oxygen to make energy, they create carbon dioxide, which must be excreted by our lungs. When the body uses protein and amino acids to build essential bodily tissues, it releases ammonia as a byproduct, which must be converted to urea by the liver, filtered by the kidneys, and excreted in the urine. Various hormones, "used" blood and immune system cells, and other wastes are excreted efficiently on a daily basis through the skin, lungs, kidneys, and bowel. Add to that the chemical cocktail of modern life, and the body's ability to cleanse itself is nothing short of miraculous!

In this section, you will learn about the body's detoxification systems and the conditions that can impair their function. After discussing the mechanics, we can then strategize ways to support the body's ability to cleanse and heal itself.

MECHANICAL SYSTEMS

The Lymphatic System

The lymphatic system is involved in the body's immune response. It consists of a collection of "drainage tubes" that collect excess fluid, waste, debris, "used" blood cells, pathogens, and toxins from the fluid that surrounds the cells in the body. Known as interstitial fluid, it contains the by-products of cellular metabolism, hormone metabolites, and immune-system components. Once collected in the lymph vessels, the fluid is called lymph, which circulates just below the skin. Eventually, lymph passes through special structures called lymph nodes and enters the blood.

The lymphatic system is passive, meaning it does not have a central "pump" like the heart, so the body relies on muscle contraction and skeletal motion to keep lymph moving for a healthy immune system. Mechanical ways to stimulate the effective flow of lymph include therapeutic massage and performing special yoga postures, or asanas. Yoga is particularly effective. The neck, groin, pelvis, and arm pits contain the greatest concentration of lymph nodes in the body, and the specific folding, bending, and twisting of certain yoga asanas compress and stretch body tissues, facilitating the release of interstitial fluids. Gentle manipulation techniques like manual lymphatic drainage, a therapy developed in Europe, can also speed the release of toxins by directing lymph to drainage sites. This is one method we routinely use in our fertility massage protocol at Pulling Down the Moon holistic fertility centers.

The Circulatory and Respiratory Systems

Once the lymph enters the blood, substances that need to be excreted can move via the circulatory system, so anything we can do to improve and strengthen circulation assists in getting rid of waste. The blood is the main route to the liver, where other metabolic byproducts and toxins are filtered out by specialized liver cells called kuppfer cells (more about this later). In our lungs excess carbon dioxide from cellular respiratory processes is released, and fresh oxygen is uploaded into circulation. The lungs, specifically our breathing patterns, can also impact body pH (acid/base balance), as well as stimulate relaxation through shifts in blood chemistry in lung capillaries.

Physical exercise, including moderate-intensity cardiovascular training and yoga, helps to strengthen the heart and improve circulation. Staying hydrated also helps support good blood volume, which can improve the body's ability to excrete toxins. Respiratory function can be improved by increased awareness of breathing patterns, by practicing breathing exercises and, of course, with cardiovascular exercise.

Integumentary System Sloughing

Toxins are also released through the skin, sweat, tears, and even the menstrual blood. So, while getting your period can be irritating—or even heartbreaking, if you are trying to conceive—rest assured that these processes help to set the stage for the renewal of body tissues.

CHEMICAL SYSTEMS

The Liver

Many toxins, both from our cellular processes (ammonia, steroid hormones) and from outside sources (drug metabolites, hormonal and other medications, and harmful environmental compounds), are removed from the blood when it flows through the liver. On a basic level, the liver acts as a filter, removing metabolic and environmental toxins and packaging them for excretion. In addition to filtering, the liver is also the site of complex chemical reactions that take toxic substances and transform them into less toxic forms that can be excreted through the urine and feces.

FILTERING: Filtering the blood is the role of kupffer cells, a type of stationary phagocyte (a.k.a. white blood cell) located in the liver. Substances filtered by the kuppfer cells include bacteria and antigens/antibodies. The kuppfer cells also remove worn-out red blood cells from circulation, conserving the iron and discarding the non-degradable portion in the form of bilirubin into the large intestine, where it is excreted as a component of feces. A liver that is sluggish or overloaded with toxins may have impaired ability to perform its filtration role, and may allow greater amounts of antigens, foreign compounds, bowel microorganisms, and other toxins to enter general circulation.

BIOTRANSFORMATION: Many toxins, including steroidal hormones and endocrine disruptors, are fat soluble and cannot enter the bloodstream for excretion via the kidneys. These substances must first be transformed into a water-soluble state through a complex chemical process that takes place in the liver. This process requires adequate protein, as well as many vitamins and minerals for optimal action. We discuss how we can use nutrition to support biotransformation in subsequent sections of this book. In addition, common-sense actions such as limiting alcohol consumption (which damages kuppfer cells) and other substances (e.g., caffeine, unnecessary medications, and recreational drugs) support liver function.

The Kidneys

The primary detoxification role of the kidneys is the production of urine. Each day our kidneys process about 200 quarts of blood and filter out two quarts of waste and excess water. The waste and water become urine, which is stored in the bladder until excretion. The kidneys are also responsible for maintaining the pH of our internal environment. Staying properly hydrated and avoiding diuretic foods and drinks is beneficial to kidney function.

THE DIGESTIVE SYSTEM

The main function of the colon (also known as the large intestine) is the storage and excretion of solid waste from the body. Most of the work of digestion and nutrient absorption occurs in the stomach and small intestines. By the time the remains of ingested food enter the colon, all that remains is the indigestible parts of foods, mostly in the form of fiber.

Digestion does occur in the colon, but not by the human body. The colon plays host to numerous colonies of bacteria that survive by breaking down these fibers for their own nourishment and in turn create usable sugars that nourish the cells of the colon. While many bacteria are beneficial and support good immune function, other less beneficial bacteria can colonize the colon. These bacteria can secrete substances that are thought to promote some cancers and may interfere with the excretion of toxins.

For optimal detoxification in the body, we want the transit time of waste in the colon to be quick, but not too quick. Constipation allows too much time for toxins to be reabsorbed into the body. On the flip side, diarrhea can damage beneficial intestinal flora, allowing less helpful bacteria to thrive.

In addition to the dietary recommendations we discuss in this book, regular physical activity and stress reduction can improve digestive health and colon function. Stress can cause diarrhea and/or constipation and may indirectly damage the intestinal flora.

MENTAL PROCESSES

The final "organ" of detoxification is actually not an organ at all—it is our ability to deal with negative thoughts and beliefs that cause emotional and physical stress. Learning to manage stress is so important, in fact, we have dedicated the entire middle section of this book to this issue. It is mindfulness, not mind, that holds the key to detoxifying our body and mind.

Mindfulness (also called Awareness) is the ability to watch the workings of our thoughts and conscious mind from the place of the witness. When we faithfully adopt the stance of mindfulness, we begin to see the patterns, and even lies, that our minds generate. When we find the space behind, between, and around our toxic mind, we find a place of infinite potential, fertility, and creativity.

So now, using our tools of awareness and proactivity, let's read on to learn how we can strengthen the body's ability to withstand the challenges around us.

CHAPTER 2

Are We Our Own Biggest Source of Toxicity?

Nine years ago, when Pulling Down the Moon integrative fertility centers first started knocking on doors and talking to physicians about holistic fertility, it was a very different world, where little, if any, credence was given to the link between lifestyle factors and fertility. Thanks to our partnerships with the medical community, and ground-breaking research from pioneers like Dr. Alice Domar in the area of mind/body medicine for fertility, the lifestyle approach to infertility has blossomed to include acupuncture, yoga, relaxation, psychotherapy, massage, and nutritional counseling.

In our opinion, the next 10 years will usher in an even greater revolution in fertility treatment, with greater emphasis on the role of lifestyle, diet, and environmental toxins as contributing factors in infertility problems. One reason for this shift is the fact that fertility patients are getting younger, making advanced maternal age a less viable "catch all" explanation for increases in the rate of infertility. Obesity, a condition associated with infertility, is also on the rise, as are sexually transmitted diseases like chlamydia that can result in infertility. Finally, environmental toxins and chemicals in our food supply are proving to be a bigger problem than we might have expected. New evidence suggests that they interfere with our hormone function, and perhaps even contribute to conditions like insulin resistance, diabetes, and obesity.

We predict that we will continue to find that the root cause of many conditions associated with infertility—including polycystic ovarian syndrome (PCOS), endometriosis, decline in egg quality, and male factor infertility—are related to oxidative stress, chronic inflammation, and impaired glucose/energy metabolism. These natural body processes can spin out of control when the body is subjected to chronic stress, poor diet, and environmental toxins.

Medical intervention for fertility, which we believe is truly amazing, is limited by its ability to treat only the symptoms of infertility, not the root causes. This is why we believe that combining lifestyle modifications and treatments, like acupuncture and traditional Chinese medicine (TCM), which address the root causes of infertility, with assisted reproductive technology (ART), will continue to prove effective and will greatly enhance the success of medical intervention.

In the gold standard of medical research—the randomized controlled clinical trial—researchers make an effort to control experimental variables so that the value of the intervention can be assessed. We would argue that perhaps the largest variable of any human trial is environment (including diet, stress levels, emotional state, exposure to toxins, and activity levels). The goal of this book is to introduce the concept of an improved *in vivo* environment—a Cleanse Lifestyle, so to speak—as the ideal state in which to conduct any fertility intervention, from low-tech "trying" to high stakes treatments like in vitro fertilization.

In this chapter, we examine specific areas of potential vulnerability that have strong connections to diet: over/underweight, insulin resistance, inflammation/oxidative stress, and poor gut health. You may wish to take notes, but it may not be necessary because at the end of this book we present a series of recommendations to help you implement the concepts discussed in depth here.

FERTILITY CHALLENGES

1. Weight: Finding (Energy) Balance

From a nutritional standpoint, the concept of Energy Balance is critical for fertility. When Energy In (the food we eat) is greater than Energy Out (our metabolism + activity), we gain weight, which can be a problem for fertility. Excess fat tissue can disrupt estrogen metabolism, and too many calories taken in can impair blood sugar regulation, with the result that overweight and obese women have a harder time getting/staying pregnant than women at a healthy body weight.

On the flip side, when Energy In is less than Energy Out, women also struggle to conceive. The body has a very precise priority for the way it uses its calories (energy). First served are the functions that are critical to life—fully functioning nervous system communication throughout the body, cellular metabolism, and respiration/circulation. Once these processes are secured, energy is diverted to less critical but still essential body functions, including locomotion, immune function, and growth. Last served are nonessential functions like reproduction, which can essentially be turned off during lean times without harming the individual. Reproductive function doesn't necessarily shut off all at once. Cycles can lengthen, the menstrual cycle can shorten, and menstruation can become scant prior to complete loss of periods.

Clearly, none of these conditions is optimal for conception. It has been estimated that problems with weight maintenance explain up to 12 percent of all cases of infertility. In terms of restoring balance and fertility in the body, getting rid of excess weight or gaining necessary weight is one of the most vital actions we can take. Since we associate fat with inactivity (think couch potato!) and fat storage, many women are surprised to learn that fat is quite metabolically active. Fat cells are major producers of the sex hormone estrogen, and while most estrogen is made by the ovaries, about 30 percent of a woman's estrogen is actually produced in her fat cells. There are three major kinds of estrogen produced within the body. Estradiol is the most potent form and is manufactured by the ovaries. Estrone, manufactured by the fat cells, is of intermediate-potency. Estriol is the weakest form of estrogen and is primarily present in the body during pregnancy.

Interestingly, a woman's body fat composition may affect the amount of estrogen circulating in her body. The steroid sex hormones estrogen and testosterone are both fat soluble and can be stored in our body's fat cells. As mentioned previously, fat cells produce estrone, a "weaker" but still metabolically active form of estrogen that has been linked to breast cancer. Estrone is also easily converted into estradiol so heavier women tend to have higher overall levels of metabolically potent estrogen than women with lower body fat (Fernandez-Real, JM et al. 1999). This excess estrogen can create hormonal imbalance in the reproductive system. Lean women have less estrogen input from fat cells. However, lean women may metabolize estrogen differently than women with excess body fat. Lean women tend to produce higher levels of 2-OH estrogen, a very weak and potentially protective form of estrogen (Sowers et al. 2006). While 2-OH estrogen may protect against cancer this form of estrogen can also create disruption in the menstrual cycle.

Our strategy for achieving optimal fertility should be to strive for an optimal body weight. Studies show a woman should aim for a Body Mass Index (BMI) of 20-25. The good news is that just a 5-10 percent decrease or increase in body weight can make a major difference in a woman's ability to conceive.

BMI and Fertility

BMI is determined by taking your weight in kilograms and dividing it by your height in meters squared.

BMI of 19–25 = Healthy
BMI 26–29 = Overweight
BMI 30–39 = Obese
BMI 40+ = Extremely Obese

Studies have shown that overweight women (BMI ≥ 26) are more likely to have ovulation problems that result in irregular or infrequent menstrual cycles and infertility. Obesity also increases the risk for ectopic pregnancies and miscarriage. With medical fertility treatment, success rates are lower in women who are overweight. This may be the result of a lower response rate to fertility medications and a higher percentage of immature eggs. (Gesink Law et al., 2007, Veleva et al., 2008).

BODY MASS INDEX MEASUREMENTS

	Normal						Overweight					Obese										Extreme Obesity														
BMI	19	20	21	22	23	24	25	26	27	28	29	30	31	32	33	34	35	36	37	38	39	40	41	42	43	44	45	46	47	48	49	50	51	52	53	54
Height (inches)																		Body Weight (pounds)																		
58	91	96	100	105	110	115	119	124	129	134	138	143	148	153	158	162	167	172	177	181	186	191	196	201	205	210	215	220	224	229	234	239	244	248	253	258
59	94	99	104	109	114	119	124	128	133	138	143	148	153	158	163	168	173	178	183	188	193	198	203	208	212	217	222	227	232	237	242	247	252	257	262	267
60	97	102	107	112	118	123	128	133	138	143	148	153	158	163	168	174	179	184	189	194	199	204	209	215	220	225	230	235	240	245	250	255	261	266	271	276
61	100	106	111	116	122	127	132	137	143	148	153	158	164	169	174	180	185	190	195	201	206	211	217	222	227	232	238	243	248	254	259	264	269	275	280	285
62	104	109	115	120	126	131	136	142	147	153	158	164	169	175	180	186	191	196	202	207	213	218	224	229	235	240	246	251	256	262	267	273	278	284	289	295
63	107	113	118	124	130	135	141	146	152	158	163	169	175	180	186	191	197	203	208	214	220	225	231	237	242	248	254	259	265	270	278	282	287	293	299	304
64	110	116	122	128	134	140	145	151	157	163	169	174	180	186	192	197	204	209	215	221	227	232	238	244	250	256	262	267	273	279	285	291	296	302	308	314
65	114	120	126	132	138	144	150	156	162	168	174	180	186	192	198	204	210	216	222	228	234	240	246	252	258	264	270	276	282	288	294	300	306	312	318	324
66	118	124	130	136	142	148	155	161	167	173	179	186	192	198	204	210	216	223	229	235	241	247	253	260	266	272	278	284	291	297	303	309	315	322	328	334
67	121	127	134	140	146	153	159	166	172	178	185	191	198	204	211	217	223	230	236	242	249	255	261	268	274	280	287	293	299	306	312	319	325	331	338	344
68	125	131	138	144	151	158	164	171	177	184	190	197	203	210	216	223	230	236	243	249	256	262	269	276	282	289	295	302	308	315	322	328	335	341	348	354
69	128	135	142	149	155	162	169	176	182	189	196	203	209	216	223	230	236	243	250	257	263	270	277	284	291	297	304	311	318	324	331	338	345	351	358	365
70	132	139	146	153	160	167	174	181	188	195	202	209	216	222	229	236	243	250	257	264	271	278	285	292	299	306	313	320	327	334	341	348	355	362	369	376
71	136	143	150	157	165	172	179	186	193	200	208	215	222	229	236	243	250	257	265	272	279	286	293	301	308	315	322	329	338	343	351	358	365	372	379	386
72	140	147	154	162	169	177	184	191	199	206	213	221	228	235	242	250	258	265	272	279	287	294	302	309	316	324	331	338	346	353	361	368	375	383	390	397
73	144	151	159	166	174	182	189	197	204	212	219	227	235	242	250	257	265	272	280	288	295	302	310	318	325	333	340	348	355	363	371	378	386	393	401	408
74	148	155	163	171	179	186	194	202	210	218	225	233	241	249	256	264	272	280	287	295	303	311	319	326	334	342	350	358	365	373	381	389	396	404	412	420
75	152	160	168	176	184	192	200	208	216	224	232	240	248	256	264	272	279	287	295	303	311	319	327	335	343	351	359	367	375	383	391	399	407	415	423	431
76	156	164	172	180	189	197	205	213	221	230	238	246	254	263	271	279	287	295	304	312	320	328	336	344	353	361	369	377	385	394	402	410	418	426	435	443

2. Blood Sugar Regulation

Typical U.S. diet % of Calories

Sugars with high glycemic load	18.6%
Refined cereal grains	20.4%

Source: Cordain et al. 2005

According to nutritional data, 39 percent of total dietary energy in the United States comes from foods that lead to insulin resistance, accompanied by high levels of blood sugar, circulating insulin, LDL ("bad") cholesterol, and triglycerides. Effective blood sugar regulation is critical for reproductive hormone balance. The reason is that our ovaries are quite sensitive to insulin, the hormone secreted by the pancreas to regulate blood sugar. When levels of insulin become higher than normal, insulin can "invade" hormone receptors on the ovaries that are designed for reproductive hormones and can disrupt communication in the control center of the endocrine system, the HPA (hypothalamic-pituitary axis). In addition, high levels of insulin cause the cells in the ovarian tissues to overproduce androgens, such as testosterone. This excess of testosterone causes the hirsutism, acne, and hair loss associated with PCOS. Hormonal dysfunction can disrupt the delicate balance of the reproductive system and make it harder for a woman to conceive.

To ensure that insulin isn't over-produced it's necessary to reduce or avoid sugary foods and processed carbohydrates (carbs) that are high on the glycemic index (high-GI foods) and favor whole, unprocessed foods that have their fiber and nutritional profile intact (low-GI foods). Unprocessed foods break down slowly in the body and produce a slow, steady stream of usable energy, avoiding the blood sugar roller coaster that leads to chronic inflammation and inflammatory conditions. The combined GI of foods that make up a meal is called its glycemic load (GL).

The impact of glycemic load on fertility was borne out by data from the famous Nurses Study 2 (Chavarro et al., 2007). In this study the quality, not the quantity, of carbohydrates a woman eats appears to be associated with ovulatory infertility. In other words, it was not the total amount of carbohydrates a woman ate that affected her ability to conceive; it was the type of carbs. Women who ate carbs that were rapidly digested ("fast" carbs), such as white bread, potatoes, and sugary foods, had higher rates of ovulatory infertility. Eating "slower" carbs—fibrous, unprocessed whole grains and fresh vegetables and fruits—was associated with lower rates of ovulatory infertility.

Studies have also shown that high blood sugar is associated with poor egg and embryo quality. The transportation of glucose, the energy source for the cells, is thought to decrease in cells consistently bathed in a high sugar environment, resulting in cell damage and death. Clearly, that's not great for fertility (Doblado et al., 2007).

Cleanse Tip: Low-Glycemic Diet

To improve fertility, we counsel our patients to closely control their blood sugar and adopt a low-glycemic dietary approach. The glycemic index (GI) is a measure of the effects of ingested carbohydrates on blood sugar levels. A food with a high glycemic score raises blood sugar amply and quickly. Lower-glycemic foods break down more slowly and release glucose into the blood more gradually. The level of processing and the amount of fiber a carbohydrate contains can affect its glycemic score. Generally, minimally processed carbs that are naturally good sources of fiber are the lowest glycemic choices.

Choosing foods strictly based on the glycemic index can actually become confusing, as many high glycemic foods are good choices because of their high nutrient density, while other foods score lower because of high fat content (i.e., carrots can score between 12 and 90 on the GI while a Snickers bar scores around 50!). Rather than get caught up in evaluating individual foods, it makes more sense to use the following tips to make your *entire dietary strategy* low-glycemic. The following guidelines will help you avoid the roller-coaster blood sugar ride that perpetuates sugar cravings and overeating.

- Avoid/eliminate highly processed, "white," and sugary foods.
- Eat regular meals and snacks; avoid long periods of fasting.
- Keep refined sugar to < 5% of total dietary calories.
- Stick to fresh fruits and vegetables and whole grain sources of carbs.
- Partner healthy fat or lean protein with carbohydrates. This will help slow the digestion and assimilation of sugars into the blood stream. Try a tablespoon of peanut or almond butter on some wheat toast, or have some guacamole with whole wheat pita chips instead of a sugary granola bar.
- Cut back on caffeinated drinks. Caffeine stimulates an immediate rise in blood sugar levels that can bring about a later crash.
- Select foods high in soluble fiber (whole grains, dried beans and peas, oat bran, barley, nuts, fruits, and vegetables) that help to control blood sugar.
- Reduce or eliminate artificial sweeteners because these are not recommended for women who are trying to conceive. Animal studies have shown the regular consumption of artificial sweeteners may lead to overeating, loss of appetite control, and weight gain (Swithers et al., 2008).

Certain supplements have been shown to help with blood sugar regulation and insulin sensitivity. One is myo-inositol, a B vitamin also used to help treat mood symptoms of PMS. Myo-inositol is the pre-metabolized form of d-chiro-inositol. Myo-inositol has been shown to improve the symptoms of PCOS, restore ovulation, and improve the quality of eggs retrieved during an IVF cycle in women with PCOS. While both d-chiro-inositol and myo-inositol have been shown to be effective for blood sugar regulation, most of the research with fertility and PCOS has been done using myo-inositol and for this reason we use myo-inositol at Pulling Down the Moon.

3. Chronic Inflammation: Another Hot Topic for Fertility

Inflammation is not a disease; it's a natural physiological process essential to our immune system and our body's ability to fight infection and heal itself. However, certain medical conditions, such as endometriosis, PCOS, pelvic inflammatory disease (PID), and premature ovarian failure, have been linked to both chronic inflammation and adverse pregnancy outcomes. Researchers hypothesize that chronic inflammation may impair the uterine environment and/or disrupt the specific chain of immune system events that allow an embryo to implant (Levin et al., 2007).

Let's begin by defining inflammation and its role in a healthy body. *Inflammation* is the body's immune response to damaged cells, infection, or allergy. *Acute inflammation* is the body's immediate response to injury or infection and is characterized by redness, heat, swelling, and pain caused by increased blood flow into the injured or infected area. In addition to increased blood flow, the acute phase of inflammation is characterized by the presence of white blood cells and phagocytes (immune cells that clean up cell damage by "eating" it). In a healthy body, acute inflammation is matched by an *anti-inflammatory* response that takes over once injury is past and promotes healing in the damaged tissues.

A condition called *chronic inflammation* results when the acute immune response remains active as a result of stress, digestive problems, environmental toxins, allergies, and other issues. In the case of chronic inflammation, pro-inflammatory immune cells continue to circulate in the body and damage healthy tissues including blood vessel linings (atherosclerosis), joint tissue (arthritis), gut mucosa (food intolerance), cell membranes and potentially reproductive cells/tissues. Inflammation is also implicated in insulin resistance, as the chemical messengers released by the immune cells of the inflammation response actually cause cells to lose their ability to respond to insulin.

PROSTAGLANDINS

The main chemical mediators of inflammation are prostaglandins, chemical messengers that turn the immune component of acute inflammation on and off. Prostaglandins are made on an as-needed basis from long-chain fatty acids present in the cells of the infected or damaged area.

There are two main groups of prostaglandins: pro-inflammatory prostaglandins (called Series 2 prostaglandins), which stimulate acute inflammation at the injury site, and the anti-inflammatory prostaglandins (called Series 1 and Series 3 prostaglandins), which turn it off.

Arachadonic acid is the main pro-inflammatory Series 2 prostaglandin active in the body. Its role is to signal the acute inflammatory response in injured cells, and it is released in the presence of injury or infection. Arachadonic acid is present in our diet in animal products (meat and dairy) and can also be manufactured from linolenic acid (also known as omega-6 fatty acids). Omega-6 fatty acids are found in corn oil, soy bean oil, and in the meat of animals that are fed corn).

ESSENTIAL FATTY ACIDS (EFAS) AND FATTY ACID COMPOSITION

On the side of the "good guys" are the omega-3 fatty acids ALA (alphalinolenic acid), found in green vegetables and grass, EPA (eicosapentaenoic acid), and DHA (docosahexaneoic acid), found in marine plants and animals. Also helpful in decreasing inflammation is gamma-linolenic acid (GLA), found in evening primrose oil. These fats provide the chemical backbone of 1- and 3-series prostaglandins that help turn off inflammation.

Chronic inflammation is a relatively new concern and is thought to be at the root of chronic health conditions like heart disease, diabetes, and cancer. Researchers hypothesize that one reason for the rise of inflammation is dietary change. The primitive human diet contained an estimated 1:1 ratio of omega-6 to omega-3 fats. Today the typical Western diet is skewed toward pro-inflammatory omega-6 fatty acids by at least 10:1 (some studies cite an astounding 20:1). Unfortunately, since the fatty acids we eat are ultimately incorporated into our tissues, this dietary shift has skewed our physiology toward inflammation.

A Natural Fire Extinguisher

Work to decrease your consumption of omega-6 fats (refined oils like corn and soy, and processed foods made with these oils) and increase your intake of omega-3s (dark leafy greens, walnuts, chia and flax seeds, cold-water fatty fish such as wild salmon, halibut, and sardines, and eggs, chicken, turkey, bison, and lean red meat beef from free-ranging grass-fed animals). The most bio-available sources of omega-3s are marine/fish oils. Unfortunately, due to environmental toxicity concerns, intake of fatty fish must be limited in women who are pregnant or trying to conceive. We do recommend a high-quality fish oil supplement that provides ample omega-3s. But just because your dad is taking 5,000 mg of fish oil a day for cardiovascular health, this doesn't mean that's right for fertility. Research in mice has shown that diets highly supplemented with omega-3s may actually increase lipid peroxidation in oocytes, which is not what we're trying to achieve! Look for a pure, quality-tested fish oil supplement that provides a daily dose of about 700 mg EPA and 500 mg DHA for a combined daily dose of 1200 mg (Wakefield, 2008).

GOOD FATS VS. BAD FATS

When it comes to fertility, fat is a very misunderstood nutrient. At the Pulling Down the Moon fertility centers, many of the women who come to us for nutritional counseling are eating a low-fat diet. This is of definite concern as eating the right amount of good fats daily is essential to fertility.

Note that data from the Nurses Study revealed that the amount of fat in the diet was *not* related to ovulatory infertility, once researchers controlled for weight, exercise, and smoking. Cholesterol, saturated fat, and monounsaturated fat did not correlate with ovulatory infertility. In addition, polyunsaturated fats were found to be loosely associated with a protective effect. The most important news from this study was this: trans fats—man-made fats used in processed foods—*were* directly linked to ovulatory infertility (Chavarro et al., 2007).

Fats fall into three major categories: saturated fat (SFAs), monounsaturated fat (MUFAs), and polyunsaturated fat (PUFAs). Monounsaturated fats have been shown to lower levels of "bad" cholesterol, protect against heart disease, and may actually aid in weight loss. Polyunsaturated fats have been shown to lower bad cholesterol as well—but not all polyunsaturated fats are beneficial. As we discuss more fully in the inflammation section of this chapter, the typical Western diet is skewed toward high intakes of omega-6 PUFAs, creating an imbalance that has dangerous consequences for heart disease, diabetes, cancer, and potentially fertility.

The amounts of monounsaturated and polyunsaturated fats we consume have implications for fertility for several reasons. First, fats are integrated into our cell membranes (including the oocyte and sperm). The health of cell membranes can have a far-reaching impact. Hormone receptors, glucose transporters, and other key regulatory proteins are "housed" in the cell membranes. Changes to the fat composition of cell membranes may actually impair the function of these transport and receptor molecules (Wathes et al., 2007). Second, healthy fats (especially fats from the omega-3 family) provide the chemical backbone for many hormones as well as anti-inflammatory components of our immune system. Finally, healthy fats support our emotional well-being and mood.

LIFESTYLE FACTORS THAT INCREASE INFLAMMATION
- Obesity
- Smoking
- Excess alcohol intake
- Stress and its hormone messenger cortisol. Cortisol raises blood sugar and insulin levels, which stimulates inflammation. In turn, inflammation impairs the ability of the cells to respond to insulin, thereby creating a vicious cycle.
- Exercise overtraining syndrome. Too much intense exercise with too little rest can create inflammation. [Angeli et al. 2004]

- Environmental toxins, including synthetic fibers, latex, glues, adhesives, plastics, air fresheners, and cleaning products that are EVERYWHERE in our environment.
- Poor dietary choices
- Food sensitivities

4. Oxidative Stress and Fertility

In common with inflammation, oxidative stress is another natural body process that is an essential part of physiological function. As we breathe and our cells produce energy, our bodies use the element oxygen and produce reactive oxygen species (commonly called free radical molecules) as a result of these normal metabolic processes. In layman's terms, we can understand ROSs, or free radicals, as highly reactive molecules that have lost an electron during a chemical reaction and roam around "stealing" electrons from other molecules. While this doesn't sound particularly scary, on a chemical level this causes a tremendous amount of trouble. This is where antioxidants enter the picture.

Antioxidants are chemical compounds that happily give up electrons to free radicals in order to keep the chemical peace. Antioxidants are present inside the body, and they also come from food. They include vitamins E, A, and C, ALA (alpha-lipoic acid) and other compounds found in fruits and vegetables, and selenium and other minerals.

As long as the levels of antioxidants in the body match ROS production, all is well. But when the balance tips, and ROS production outstrips antioxidant ability, free radicals begin to wreak havoc on DNA, cell membranes, and tissues. This condition is called oxidative stress (OS), and it can cause damage to the lipid membranes of cells in the body, alter protein and DNA, and cause cell death. OS is implicated in chronic diseases like cancer and heart disease.

The relationship between oxidative stress and male fertility is fairly well established. Sperm-related dysfunctions associated with oxidative stress include low sperm count, poor sperm motility, and problems with sperm-oocyte fusion (Fraczek M et al. 2007). In terms of female fertility, studies have shown that poor antioxidant status and high levels of free radicals are associated with endometriosis, PCOS, decline in ovarian function, and poor IVF outcomes (Ruder et al., 2008).

Antioxidants and Fertility: Beyond A, C, and E—CoQ10 and Oxidative Stress

Researchers in Toronto are exploring a hypothesis that oxidative stress is a major player in the decline of egg quality seen with age, and they are testing whether supplementation with the mitochondrial nutrient CoEnzymeQ10 can reverse this damage.

The process of egg maturation and ovulation is incredibly energy intensive. All the "fuel" for the egg is provided by mitochondria, the energy powerhouses inside the cells where chemical energy is produced. Eggs have the most mitochondria of any cell in the body—more than even energy-guzzling muscle and nerve cells. The huge energy needs of the oocytes is due to the fact that the egg must divide its genetic material at least once with ovulation, and then a second time if fertilized. This process of splitting off and extruding chromosomes is wildly energy intensive. To accomplish this feat, the oocyte must actually increase the mitochondria mass 40-fold during follicle recruitment.

The result of this massive works project is a loss of mitochondrial function due to the accumulation of mutations. This impairs the ability of the egg to split the genetic material—a result that may increase the rates of genetic abnormalities found in the offspring of older women. It may also explain the poor survival rate of embryos from older women. CoQ10 is a not a vitamin; it is a fat-soluble substance found in almost all cell membranes. It is a key component in the process of making cellular energy and also serves as a powerful antioxidant. Our body tissues make CoQ10, but levels decline with age. Studies have shown supplementation with CoQ10 may improve many diseases (hypertension, congestive heart failure, Parkinson's disease, and poor sperm motility). Now scientists have shown the beneficial impact of CoQ10 supplementation on egg and embryo quality in both rats and cows. A new study [Bentov et al.] is following the outcome of supplementation with 600 mg of CoQ10 in older women undergoing fertility treatment with the aim of improving egg quality by bolstering mitochondrial function.

GLUTATHIONE: ROLES IN ENERGY PRODUCTION AND DETOXIFICATION

Glutathione, a combination of the amino acids gamma-glutamic acid, cysteine, and glycine, is arguably our body's most important cellular antioxidant (Wu et al., 2004). Glutathione is present in the cell matrix, including the mitochondria and nucleus. The liver is the biggest producer of glutathione. Some of its many roles in the body include:

- Directly scavenging reactive oxygen species, or free radicals, that can damage cell DNA
- Reacting with intermediate metabolites of toxins—notably estrogen—and facilitating their conversion to water-soluble substances that can be excreted in urine
- Contributing to spermatogenesis and sperm maturation

Clearly, maintaining healthy levels of glutathione is important for minimizing oxidative stress in the body and getting rid of excess estrogens and other hormone-mimicking compounds. Unlike other antioxidants, oral supplementation with glutathione is not effective. The best strategy for supporting glutathione activity in the body is to ensure ample consumption of foods important to glutathione synthesis. Foods like asparagus, broccoli, avocado, and spinach are associated with elevating glutathione status, as well as foods high in the sulfur-containing amino acids cysteine (found in high-protein food like chicken, cottage cheese, and oats) and methionine (found in meat, fish, beans, garlic, and lentils). Other important nutrients for glutathione metabolism include the mineral selenium and the B-vitamin riboflavin.

FLAVONOIDS

Flavonoids are bioactive substances that create the beautiful color in plants. When consumed as part of the human diet, these compounds serve as antioxidants. Examples of flavonoids include resveratrol, the pigment present in grape skins that has become famous for its anti-aging properties, and the catechins that make green tea such an effective antioxidant.

DIETARY RECOMMENDATIONS FOR IMPROVING ANTIOXIDANT STATUS

The following lifestyle/nutrition behaviors will limit your exposure to oxidative stress:
- Quit smoking.
- Limit alcohol consumption.
- Provide your body ample time for rest and recovery after exercise — don't overtrain.
- Manage your stress.

Increase your body's antioxidant capacity by eating a MINIMUM of three servings of vegetables per day and at least two servings of fruit. Where possible we highly encourage the consumption of organic produce. Save money with a simple rule - if a vegetable or fruit has a thick and inedible skin (think winter squash, oranges and bananas) you do not need to spend money for organic. Another good guideline is the color rule: choose an orange, a green, and a yellow vegetable every day to ensure you're getting a variety of flavonoids as well as a wide array of vitamins and minerals. This is sometimes called "eating the rainbow."

Ensure an adequate protein intake that includes good sources of the sulfur-containing amino acids methionine and glycine: meat, fish, beans, and lentils.

5. Gut Function and Fertility

Gut flora, or friendly bacteria, have multiple functions in a healthy digestive system, including the following:
- Assisting with the digestion of fiber and other carbohydrates in the colon that feed both the host (human) and the beneficial bacteria
- Helping with the metabolism and absorption of vitamin K, iron, and magnesium
- Keeping out bad bacteria that would otherwise invade the body

But now it seems that these tiny, one-celled creatures may be able to "play stork." Researchers have found a connection between bacterial vaginosis (BV) and a range of adverse pregnancy outcomes ranging from miscarriage to preterm birth. These researchers hypothesize vaginosis may also be implicated in some cases of IVF failure, as higher than normal rates of BV are found in IVF patients (Verstraelen et al. 2005). Healthy levels of gut flora may stop the development of bacterial vaginosis.

Other research suggests that intestinal flora can prevent early pregnancy loss. Two potential mechanisms are outlined. In the first scenario, direct migration of bacteria from a compromised area into the uterus causes inflammation and potentially an immune response against the developing embryo. In the second scenario, chemical signals from the compromised gut stimulate a generalized inflammation response that interferes with implantation and/or early development of the fetus (Friebe et al 2008). Both groups suggest that dietary changes and supplementation with probiotics may improve IVF and pregnancy success and should be considered as a potential avenue for treatment.

DIETARY RECOMMENDATIONS TO SUPPORT FRIENDLY GUT BACTERIA

1. Supplement your diet with high-quality probiotics.
2. Include soluble fiber (oatmeal, chia seeds, beans, and lentils) and complex carbohydrates, which are the preferred foods of beneficial bacteria, in your diet. Gut bacteria munch on fiber residue and manufacture short-chain fatty acids and vitamins that maintain colon health.
3. Do not eat excessive amounts of red meat because it can produce excess sulfur, which promotes the growth of sulfur-metabolizing flora and increases the production of carcinogens.
4. Limit sugar and fat in the diet in order to cut down on hostile bacteria.

Surprise "Players" in the Hormone Equation:
Beneficial Gut Bacteria and Glucose and Estrogen Metabolism

New research is pointing to some unexpected "soldiers" in the battle for good blood sugar and hormone health. Experimental evidence has shown that diets enhanced with probiotics (beneficial gut bacteria) have a positive effect on glucose metabolism in mice. Recently, research in women has also found that the combination of probiotic supplementation and dietary counseling led to better glucose metabolism than was the case with dietary counseling alone during pregnancy (Laitinen et al. 2005) . The mechanism of action is not yet well understood, but researchers hypothesize that beneficial gut bugs accomplish the following:

- Limit the proliferation of other "bad" bacteria that can break down starches in the large intestine that would otherwise be excreted. The breakdown of these starches by the bad bugs into sugars increases the glucose load to our body
- Improve gut immunity and limit inflammatory action, which has been associated with insulin resistance and obesity

The beneficial bacteria in our gut also play an important role in the excretion of estrogen metabolites and hormone-like environmental toxins. When beneficial bacteria are in good supply, the elimination of waste is speedy and regular and estrogen is excreted quickly. However, when good gut bacteria is compromised due to inflammation, allergy, antibiotics, or other conditions, bad intestinal bacteria begin to thrive. These less friendly critters secrete the enzyme β-glucuronidase, which redigests estrogen in the large intestines, releasing it back into the body. High levels of β-glucuronidase are associated with breast and colon cancer and may contribute to hormone imbalances associated with infertility.

6. Food Sensitivity and Fertility

You may find it surprising to learn that your digestive system is part of your immune system, but the gut actually functions as the body's first line of defense, eliminating bacteria and other bugs before they can infect our internal environment. When the digestive system is challenged by such conditions as stress, illness, or food sensitivity, inflammation can occur as a result of adrenal stress hormones being secreted to manage the impacts.

Frequent bouts of diarrhea, constipation, intestinal bloating/cramping, and heartburn may all be signs of an inflamed digestive tract. Chronic inflammation in the digestive tract can impair the body's ability to break down and absorb the nutrients in the food we eat. In addition, gut inflammation may affect other organ systems, including the reproductive organs, which are in close proximity. These factors, taken together, are why we take a very close look at digestion and symptoms of food sensitivity, as they relate to fertility when patients attend our fertility centers.

The classic example of the connection between food sensitivity and infertility is celiac disease, a condition in which an individual cannot tolerate gluten (a protein found naturally in wheat and used as an additive in many foods). Recent studies show that celiac disease affects about 1 percent of the US population, and the condition often goes undiagnosed (Evans et al., 2009). It is estimated that 4.8 percent of U.S. women with undiagnosed infertility suffer from celiac disease, and men with celiac disease also have a higher risk of subfertility and impotence.

While the mechanism by which celiac disease impairs fertility is not fully understood, scientists have made educated guesses as to the link. Celiac disease is autoimmune in nature.

If an individual is genetically predisposed to celiac disease, dietary intake of gluten (a protein found in many grains) causes a two-fold attack in the small intestine. Antibodies first attack the gluten protein, and this attack triggers an autoimmune response in which antibodies attack the smooth muscle component in the small intestine, damaging the *villi* (tiny, fingerlike protrusions on the wall of the small intestine that absorb nutrients from food). This points to the most likely link between celiac disease and infertility: the malabsorption of nutrients, in particular iron and folic acid. Iron deficiency can lead to anemia (a condition that is common in persons with celiac disease). Iron deficiency has recently been implicated in ovulatory infertility, and iron-containing proteins play an important role in the release and transport of the egg at the time of ovulation.

Researchers are now hypothesizing that even in the absence of full-blown celiac disease, gluten sensitivity can cause symptoms similar to inflammatory bowel disease, which may negatively impact nutrition status and quality of life in ways similar to celiac disease (Verdu et al., 2009).

Other common food sensitivities include eggs, soy, peanuts, and dairy. Symptoms of food sensitivity are diverse: diarrhea, constipation, rashes, gas, bloating, and headaches—to name a few. At Pulling Down the Moon, in cases of repeated miscarriage, multiple failed assisted reproduction technology cycles, and unexplained infertility, our nutritionists often choose to eliminate these common allergens from the diet and track any change in digestive function and other symptoms. Please note, though, that the elimination of any food from the diet requires careful nutritional planning and should not be undertaken without help from a nutritionist. Elimination diets, if done improperly, can mask serious problems like celiac disease, which may require further intervention.

CHAPTER 3

Challenges from the Environment

In the previous chapter we examined how a healthy diet can limit toxicity by reducing the negative impact of overweight and insulin resistance, inflammation, oxidative stress, and poor gut function. No matter how healthy our diet, however, challenges from the environment remain. It's a double-edged sword, really. Many of the scientific advances that have extended and improved our quality of life—from factory farming to the hormone treatment of livestock as well as pharmacology and industrial chemistry—have have also increased the chemical load our bodies must manage.

The good news is that this story, which seems so modern, is actually quite ancient. Animal/plant warfare has been with us from the beginning of life on earth, when plants synthesized chemicals to deter animals from eating them, and animals subsequently evolved mechanisms for removing these chemicals from their bodies. The complexity of modern life has thickened the plot, but the essential message—that our bodies are designed to cope with these substances—remains. That's not to say that we should kick back, relax, and shovel in the chemicals, but we do not have to panic.

Spoiler alert: The first part of this chapter is a total downer. As is required in any book that purports to discuss toxicity and fertility, we've included a laundry list of the most common sources of toxic exposure, so you can learn a bit more about chemicals that impact fertility. The second part of the chapter outlines strategies for limiting exposure to harmful substances. Finally, we explore ways of supporting our body's natural detoxification pathways.

CHEMICALS AND FOOD ADDITIVES

The food we eat is one of the most obvious places that foreign substances enter our bodies. Preservatives, artificial colors and flavors, and hormones are the most common sources of xenobiotics (a fancy word for a chemical found in an organism that is not made by the organism). Let's take a closer look at these categories now.

Artificial Flavors and Color

While generally recognized as safe, the data on artificial flavors and colors are sufficiently inconclusive to recommend eliminating these substances from the body. From our perspective, the rationale for limiting consumption of these additives is straightforward; it doesn't even rely on scientific data. Foods that contain artificial colors and flavors are usually over-processed and have empty nutritional value (candy, pop, frozen dinners). This simple commitment to avoiding artificial colors and flavors will steer you toward nutrient rich and health-affirming foods.

Hormones in Our Food Supply

Hormones and hormone-like substances are present in our food supply. They enter through meat, dairy, and plant sources. While not overtly toxic, these substances can mimic the action of our own sex hormones and have the potential to interfere with reproduction.

Meat

The Nurses Study found ovulatory infertility to be most prevalent in women with the highest protein intakes. In addition, women who ate more vegetable protein seemed to have a lower incidence of ovulation problems. At Pulling Down the Moon, we do encourage the intake of some animal protein when a woman is trying to conceive. Rather than factory-farmed meats, we suggest free-range, grass-fed poultry and game meats like bison and venison. The forage-fed diet of these animals tends to create leaner meat with a healthier fat profile. They are also not subject to hormone treatment aimed at controlling disease, which is necessary when huge numbers of animals are raised in factory conditions in feedlots. In terms of vegetable protein, we tend to stay away from large amounts of soy (see below), but we do encourage a daily serving of beans or lentils as part of a woman's protein intake.

Phytoestrogens

Phytoestrogens are substances found in plants that act as weak estrogens in our bodies. Common dietary sources of phytoestrogens include soy, flax and chia seeds, kudzu, and clover.

The jury is still out when it comes to phytoestrogens and fertility because the phytoestrogen/fertility connection has not yet been thoroughly investigated. One recent study found that soy consumption in men was associated with low sperm concentration (Chavarro et al. 2008). In addition, a limited number of food studies on women have shown that diets high in soy can lower ovarian hormone levels—something that may not be good for some infertility diagnoses but could be beneficial for others (Cassidy et al., 1994, Lu et al., 2001, Lu J, et al., 1996).

Two studies have looked at supplementation with phytoestrogens during medical fertility treatment. One investigation supplemented the follicular phase (days 1-12) of clomid cycles with the herb black cohosh. This phytoestrogen treatment resulted in thicker endometrial linings and higher pregnancy rates. The rate of pregnancy was 36.7 percent in the phytoestrogen group versus 13.6 percent in the clomid-only group (Shahin et al., 2008). The second study administered soy isoflavones along with progesterone during the second-half of IVF cycles (postembryo transfer) and noted significant improvements in endometrial thickness and both clinical and ongoing pregnancy rates (Unfer et al, 2004).

Soy

At Pulling Down the Moon, we recommend that women and men limit their dietary intake of soy to no more than one 8-oz serving per day and that any soy consumed be eaten in a fermented form, such as miso, tofu, tempeh, natto, and so forth. Soy contains high amounts of phytic acid, a compound that binds iron, copper, magnesium, calcium, and zinc in the digestive tract and blocks their absorption. Soy can also be difficult to digest and can cause bloating, gas, and other gastrointestinal problems. Societies that consume soy as part of their traditional diet, such as Japan, know that it takes more than "ordinary" cooking to make soy more digestible. When soy is fermented, it is predigested by bacteria, which makes it easier to digest and removes the phytic acid.

We also recommend that you avoid processed forms of soy like soy milk, textured vegetable protein (TVP), and other "mock-meats." To make the soy in these foods digestible, they are chemically and mechanically treated to make fractured soy isolate proteins. You can identify these processed forms of soy on labels as "soy protein isolate" and "soy protein concentrate." In addition, we do not recommend supplementation with soy isoflavones or the consumption of energy bars, drinks, or shakes that contain added phytoestrogens. We also suggest avoiding genetically-modified soy products (GMO-soy) for reasons we discuss below.

Flax

Flaxseeds contain lignans (not to be confused with lignins, the insoluble fiber substance found in root vegetables, fruits like strawberries that have edible seeds and in the outer layer of grains) that are converted to powerful phytoestrogens by intestinal bacteria. In addition, flaxseed is a rich source of the omega-3 fatty acid ALA (alpha-linolenic acid), which is a precursor to the essential fatty acids EPA and DHA (see chapter 2). Flaxseed oil is sold as a health food, but we do not recommend its use. Flax oil is highly unsaturated and subject to oxidation. If you consume flax, do so moderately, no more than one tablespoon per day, since flax, like soy beans, contains high amounts of phytic acid and potentially bio-active phytoestrogens. Flax seed and flax seed oil should be refrigerated to avoid spoilage.

Other Phytoestrogens

Phytoestrogen supplements that claim to help balance hormones, improve menopausal symptoms, and cure PMS abound in the marketplace. Substances in these products include flax and soy, as well as other plant compounds high in phytoestrogens like clover, kudzu, and black cohosh. We do not recommend supplementation with any phytoestrogen products, unless you are under the supervision of a nutritionist who specializes in fertility. At Pulling Down the Moon, we do use short-term supplementation with non-soy phytoestrogens in cases in which excess estrogen may be part of the root cause of infertility (endometriosis, fibroids, obesity), or after a failed assisted reproductive technology cycle or miscarriage. This treatment is part of a fertility-specific program and is *never* combined with or used during ART treatment.

Dairy

Using the same hormone-free philosophy as we take with soy, we recommend limiting dairy consumption to one serving a day. In addition to containing added growth hormones (unless labeled as non rBGH), the milk we drink today also contains the naturally present reproductive hormones of the female cow at higher levels than in years past.

A recent review of clinical evidence linking consumption of cow's milk with higher incidence of hormone-related cancers led researchers to point a finger toward the modern agribusiness practice of milking pregnant cows. According to this review, milk from a pregnant cow can contain up to 33 percent more estrogen than milk from a cow that is not pregnant (Ganmaa D. et al., 2005). Another group of researchers compared levels of estrogen in raw and processed milk from non-pregnant and pregnant cows and found the lowest levels of estrogens in raw milk from non-pregnant cows. The highest levels came from the milk of pregnant cows. The level of estrogen in processed milk, which generally contains a blend of milk from pregnant and non-pregnant cows, was on a par with raw milk from cows in the first and second trimester of pregnancy.

The researchers concluded that a person's daily intake of estrogen from milk is "dramatically more than currently recognized." (Malekinejad H. et al., 2006). Because the jury is still out on this topic, we recommend limiting the amount of dairy consumed as part of your fertility diet to one 8-oz serving per day. We also recommend that this serving come from full-fat (whole milk) dairy, as the consumption of full-fat dairy may be protective against ovulatory infertility. Full-fat dairy also contains less of the bioactive substance IGF-1, which has been linked to cancer, acne, and other hormone-related conditions. Of course, if you limit the amount of dairy you consume, you need to ensure that you are consuming adequate amounts of calcium from other dietary sources.

Genetically Modified Organisms (GMO) in the Food Supply

Genetically modified organisms are an emerging area of concern for overall health and, specifically, fertility. GMO grains have been modified to tolerate pesticides and/or produce insecticide toxins from genetic material that has been inserted into their genome via "transgenes." Commercial GMO crops have been shown to contain pesticide residues of endocrine-disrupting chemicals at levels as high as 1000 times the amount shown to exert measurable biological effects. Until further trans-generational studies are conducted on the safety of GMO's we recommend, where possible, buying foods that are "GMO-free" (Spirous de Vendomis, J. et al., 2010).

Alcohol

The relationship between alcohol intake and infertility is still somewhat unclear. The Nurses Study did not find any association between alcohol intake and ovulatory infertility (Chavarro et al., 2009). However, studies have also shown a link between alcohol and infertility, especially IVF failure, when a woman consumes more than four drinks per week (Rossi et al., 2011). There may be some mechanism at work that makes subfertile women and couples more susceptible to the negative effects of alcohol on fertility.

Alcohol is often called an antinutrient because of its high caloric value and low nutritional value. In high levels, alcohol can actually overwhelm the liver, the body's main detox organ, and result in the creation of toxic byproducts that can severely damage bodily tissues and increase oxidative stress. Alcohol can also deplete essential nutrients and has been shown to interfere with folate absorption and metabolism, as well as folate storage in the liver. Vitamin B12 and vitamin A status can also be impaired by even moderate alcohol intake. Essential minerals like calcium are also affected by alcohol. Calcium is lost in greater quantities in the urine when alcohol is consumed.

In terms of fertility, limiting alcohol intake to fewer than three drinks per week and eliminating alcohol for one month prior to and during your IVF cycle is a prudent approach. If you do choose to drink alcohol, you may want to try an alcoholic beverage, like red wine or a dark beer, which may confer some antioxidant and cardiovascular benefits.

Caffeine

Caffeine is both a stimulant and an antidepressant. In terms of fertility, the data surrounding caffeine suggests that intakes of less than 50 mg per day do not seem to impact a woman's ability to conceive. From a holistic point of view, the need for a caffeinated "pick-me-up" may suggest that other elements in life are out of balance (poor sleep quality, peaks and valleys in blood sugar, lack of exercise) so our preference would be the elimination of caffeine from the diet. However, we can be reasonable. Our recommendation is that you reduce your caffeine intake to less than 50 mg per day.

ENVIRONMENTAL CONTAMINANTS

Cigarette Smoke

Quitting smoking is a no-brainer for fertility and detoxification. Smoking is strongly associated with infertility. There are many reasons why this may be so, including increased levels of oxidative stress and toxic chemicals in the smoke. A new study also found that women who smoked had higher levels of FSH during the first half of the menstrual cycle and higher levels of LH during the second half of the menstrual cycle, which suggests that the ovaries are not as responsive to reproductive hormones in women who smoke (Whitcomb et al., 2010). In another recent study on the impact of smoking, alcohol, and caffeine on indicators of ovarian age, only smoking was associated with high FSH, an indicator of ovarian age and poor egg quality (Kinney et al., 2007). Bottom line: Don't smoke!

Marijuana and Other Controlled Substances

Don't smoke pot, either. Or do drugs. More and more research supports the view that marijuana impairs both male and female fertility. Women who regularly smoke pot have disrupted menses, suppressed egg production, and poor embryo development. Male regular marijuana smokers experience ejaculation problems, poor sperm count and motility, and loss of libido/impotence—not to mention a severe case of the munchies (Bari et al., 2011).

Persistent Organic Pollutants

Persistent Organic Pollutants (POPs) are compounds in our environment that do not degrade and as such have the potential to bioaccumulate in animal and human tissue. POPs include some pesticides, solvents, plastic, and pharmaceuticals—all substances that have been introduced both intentionally and unintentionally into our environment by humans. Other contaminants include heavy metals like lead and mercury that are present in exhaust fumes and can bio-accumulate in the plants and animals that form our food chain. The American Society for Reproductive Medicine published a review of the science linking environmental contaminants with female infertility and found the strongest link between lead and adverse reproductive outcomes, followed by exposure to endocrine-disrupting chemicals in pesticides and POPs (Mendola et al., 2008). In a similar review of environmental contaminants and male fertility, researchers found links between exposure to chemicals like bisphenol A and phthalates and male infertility (Hauser et al., 2008).

Pesticides

Many of the chemicals used to keep pests away from food crops actually fall into the category of endocrine disruptors. For this reason we recommend that when possible, women who are trying to conceive and to minimize exposure to environmental contaminants choose certified organic produce. Conventional (nonorganic) foods may contain traces of chemical fertilizers, insecticides, and herbicides. Conventionally raised livestock and poultry may have been given antibiotics, growth hormones, and medications to accelerate growth and prevent disease. Organic products use natural fertilizers like compost or manure, beneficial insects to control pests, and manage weeds through crop rotation, weeding, and mulching. Organically raised animals are provided organic feed and have access to the outdoors. Methods like grazing, free-range diet, and clean living conditions are used to promote optimal health and growth. For a product to carry the USDA Certified Organic seal, it must be at least 95 percent organic.

Endocrine Disruptors

Of particular concern for fertility is a family of toxins called endocrine disruptors. According to the National Institute of Environmental Health Sciences, endocrine disruptors are substances that interfere with our body's hormonal systems and cause adverse developmental, reproductive, neurological, and immune effects in humans and wildlife. They are associated with infertility and cancer, as well as developmental problems. Endocrine disruptors are found in many places, including pesticides, plastics, industrial byproducts, building materials, and pollution. Unlike other toxins, even in minute concentrations, endocrine disruptors have a powerful effect on physiology. Common endocrine disrupting chemicals include:

- DDT is perhaps the most infamous and well-known endocrine disruptor. Now banned in many countries, DDT was first used to control insects in commercial crops and was later used to control pest-borne illness during World War II. DDT was later found to have disastrous effects on wildlife, and current research suggests it can impair female reproductive development. The chemical is still used in Africa and parts of Southeast Asia to control malaria, and a correlation between exposure to DDT and menstrual cycle disruption has been found in women from this area (Windham et al., 2005).

  Banned in 1977, PCBs (polychlorinated biphenyls) are found in industrial coolants and lubricants. These chemicals cause both acute and chronic health problems, including cancer and negative effects on the immune, reproductive, nervous, and endocrine systems. While these chemicals are no longer produced, they can leak into the environment from toxic waste sites, disposal of PCB wastes, and accumulation in the food chain.

- BISPHENOL A, commonly called BPA, is a component of plastic found in water bottles, baby bottles, toys, and dental appliances. Concern about BPA stems from its similarity to estrogen and its ability to bind to estrogen receptors in the human body. BPA has been shown to disrupt endocrine and fertility function in animals and is linked to risk of infertility and miscarriage in humans (Foster et al., 2008)

- **PHTHALATES** are chemicals added to plastics to make them more flexible, and phthalate compounds are also found in personal care products such as cosmetics, skin- and hair-care products, perfumes and aromatherapy products, and sex toys made of "jelly rubber." Certain phthalates have been shown to disrupt endocrine function and fertility in animals, and urinary levels of phthalates are associated with male infertility (Hauser et al., 2008). Common names of phthalate esters include di-2-ethyl hexyl phthalate (DEHP), diisodecyl phthalate (DIDP), and diisononyl phthalate (DINP).

Heavy Metals

Small amounts of heavy metals (chemical elements with specific gravity at least five times that of water) are common in our environment and diet, and tiny amounts of these metals are necessary for good health. However, when we are acutely or chronically exposed to higher levels of heavy metals, serious health consequences can result. Heavy metals are implicated in organ damage, mental and central nervous system damage, and potentially infertility. Heavy metals of concern include arsenic, lead, cadmium, mercury, and aluminum.

In particular, heavy metals are associated with oxidative stress and may also impair mitochondrial function (energy metabolism) in the cells. Our bodies use specific proteins, called metallothioneins, to bind and transport heavy metals to the liver, where they are conjugated to glutathione and excreted into the bile and feces. When we support the body's production of metallothioneins, we support its ability to bind and excrete heavy metals. Foods rich in the sulfur-containing amino acids methionine and cysteine, as well as foods rich in the mineral zinc, can increase the body's production of metallothioneins.

Polycyclic Aromatic Hydrocarbons (PAHs)

Recent headlines have been screaming about the extinction of humankind due to declining sperm quality. It is becoming an epidemic, sources say, due to environmental concerns, including the consumption of polycyclic aromatic hydrocarbons (PAHs), chemicals considered to be "genotoxic," or highly damaging to our genetic material. Studies have shown that higher levels of PAHs in the urine are associated with poor sperm quality and cancer in men (Xia et al., 2009).

Most PAHs arise from man-made sources—auto exhaust, chemical sludge, industrial plants, wood-burning stoves, oil contamination of surface water, and smoke (forest fire, waste incineration, and cigarettes)—that make their way into the food chain through bioaccumulation. Soil and crops grown near motorways have higher concentrations of PAHs. And, because PAHs are fat-soluble, they are stored in the fat tissue of plants and animals. Grazing animals, such as poultry and cattle, are particularly susceptible to PAHs, since they consume both vegetation and particulate matter from the soil. PAH-contaminated soil also washes into rivers and oceans, where filtering animals, such as mussels and oysters, become contaminated. Unfortunately there's another common way to create PAHs—and that's on the barbie. Meat, including fish and poultry, but especially red meat, contains amino acids, sugars, and a protein called creatinine that combine to form PAHs when it is heated to a very high temperature. Grilling is one of the few cooking techniques that create the kind of heat necessary for the formation of PAHs.

Grilled Meats

At our house we've even got a name for the team of carnivorous males who gather around the grill with cold beers and tongs while the meat cooks—the Torch Brothers. The tie that binds these brothers is not a tie of blood, but rather one of sizzling fat and grill tools. Apart from the "testosterone fumes" that drift in from the patio, we've always assumed these male-bonding moments are harmless ... and someone besides us is doing the cooking. How could this be a bad thing?

Unfortunately, grilled meats are a significant source of PAHs. But a world without men (and a summer without burgers) is a bleak world indeed. Is it possible to enjoy a cookout without endangering the health of our hubbies and future male children? As always, the key is moderation and intelligence (arguably not qualities found in high concentration in the Torch Brethren). So here is some important info to pass along to the boys out back:

1. Use moderation. Grilling once a week (with good grill techniques) is fine but not every night.
2. Choose lean meats and trim excess fat from meat *before* it hits the grill.
3. Avoid "flame-ups." When fat drips onto hot coals, PAHs are formed, and the resulting vapor is reabsorbed by the meat like a toxic steam bath.
4. Discard charred meats. Where you see black and burnt, PAHs have been released and reabsorbed. We repeat: charred is a bad thing.
5. Serve fresh, raw vegetables on the side of your grilled meal. The antioxidants in fresh vegetables combat DNA damage from PAHs.
6. Top your burger with onions. At least one study in mice (Izawa H. et al, 2008) shows that onions (especially red onions) contain a compound called quercetin that may protect sperm damage by PAHs. So add the onions ... just don't grill them.
7. Avoid grilling cured meats that contain nitrates and liquid smoke products.
8. Limit PAH consumption from other sources: Don't smoke; wash the waxy surface of vegetables very thoroughly; if you burn wood in your fireplace, make sure you've got good ventilation.

POPs, PAHS, and Heavy Metals as "Obesogens"

As if the disruption of our endocrine signaling weren't enough, new clinical evidence suggests even more pernicious effects of POPs—the uncoupling of energy metabolism reactions resulting in a tendency toward overweight and obesity. Estrogen plays an important role in regulating the body's management of glucose and fat, as well as the actual "energy powerhouses" of the cells, the mitochondria. It is now hypothesized that endocrine-disrupting chemicals may be interfering with estrogen's role in energy management and making it harder for our bodies to burn calories. Yikes! (Chen et al., 2009).

Simple Steps for Limiting Environmental Contaminant Exposure

1. Read ingredient labels. Look for common acronyms DBP and DEP, which are in personal care products like nail polishes, deodorants, and colognes. DHEP is found in plastics, and DMP is commonly used in insect repellent and some plastics.
2. Obviously, phthalate-free is a good thing!
3. When a product lists "fragrance," be wary, as this is often a phrase used to denote a cocktail of compounds that may contain phthalates.
4. Look at the recycling code. Plastics coded 1, 2, or 5 (the most frequently recycled) are less likely to contain phthalates and BPA. Plastics coded 3 and 7 are more likely to contain these compounds.
5. Limit exposure to BPA by limiting your consumption of canned foods.
6. Avoid plastic water bottles and use only BPA-free plastics. Warning: studies show that even BPA-free water bottles may still contain harmful chemicals.
7. Choose organically raised produce when possible. Wash fruits and vegetables thoroughly.
8. To reduce exposure to heavy metals, think twice about products you may be using that contain heavy metals: fertilizers, fungicides, insect/rodent poisons, lead-based paint, hobby supplies, furniture refinishing chemicals, and the like. Take precautions to decontaminate skin, clothing, and hair after work or hobby exposure to heavy metals.
9. Avoid fish that tend to be heavy sources of toxic metals (a full list is included in Section 3).

IT'S NOT ALL GLOOM AND DOOM

Okay, so by this point in the chapter, you may be feeling that the cards are stacked against healthy living and optimal fertility. But again, the message is not one of doom. Remember the concept of plant/animal warfare we mentioned earlier. The human body has evolved an amazing ability to cope with foreign substances. In the first chapter of this book, we looked at all the different detoxification systems our bodies use to manage endotoxins (byproducts of metabolism, bacterial byproducts) and exotoxins (drugs, environmental chemicals). In this section, it is time to look a bit closer at one specific organ, the liver, and its role in handling potentially toxic compounds on a chemical level and how our food choices support these efforts.

As Julia Child Might Say ... Save the Liver!

In terms of managing foreign substances, our liver is the epicenter of detox activity. On a mechanical level, the liver serves as a filter—pulling microbes and other waste out of our blood. On a chemical level, the liver is the site of a series of complex chemical reactions—known as biotransformation reactions—that allow the body to get rid of chemical, hormonal, and other waste that could otherwise build up and become harmful. Most of what is known about biotransformation comes from researchers in the field of pharmacology and the study of drug clearance, but these actions are also important for the clearance of hormones and environmental contaminants.

Many drugs, environmental chemicals, and hormones are lipophilic, which means they are attracted to our body's fatty tissues and could, without intervention, remain in our bodies for years. For lipophilic substances to be excreted from the body, they must first be pulled from circulation and made water-soluble so they can leave the body through our kidneys and bowel. Biotransformation occurs in two steps, called Phase 1 and Phase 2.

In Phase 1, the drug or hormone is made water-soluble by the addition of a chemical group that is water friendly. Unfortunately this water-friendly intermediate molecule is often highly reactive and potentially more "toxic" to body tissues. In Phase 2 reactions, this reactive intermediary is further processed and hooked to another chemical group that makes the molecule less reactive and more easily excreted (Grant et al., 1991).

Interestingly, many of the enzymes and essential co-factors (chemical helpers) in these important reactions come from the diet—including amino acids and the vitamins and minerals found in fruits and vegetables. As we take a closer look at the biotransformation of estrogen and estrogen-like substances in the liver, we can better understand the link between diet and detox processes and how we can eat to support the liver's efforts. At least one study has found an association between impaired liver detoxification enzymes and recurrent miscarriage. The researchers suggest that impaired biotransformation function may lead to reproductive toxicity and result in endometriosis, miscarriage, and poor pregnancy outcome (Parveen et al., 2010).

Estrogen Metabolism: An Example of Biotransformation

Imbalances in estrogen metabolism have been linked to infertility-related conditions including endometriosis, uterine fibroids, and PCOS. Lifetime exposure to estrogens has also been accepted as a risk for breast cancer. What is now becoming clear is that intermediaries of estrogen metabolism can also be viewed as a potential health hazard.

PHASE 1 BIOTRANSFORMATION: The lion's share of estrogen metabolism takes place in the liver, where it is processed for excretion in urine and feces. The first step is hydroxylation, where a water-soluble chemical group is attached to the estrogen molecule. This group can attach at one of three places: 2OH, 16OH, or 4OH. The 2OH metabolite is weak and can only form a loose bond with estrogen receptors and as such 2OH metabolites may actually be anti-estrogenic in action. The 16OH and 4OH metabolites are not so beneficial. They continue estrogenic activity and have the ability to promote cellular growth and exert estrogen-like effects. In fact, the urinary ratio of 16OH/2OH estrogen has been proposed as a predictor of breast cancer risk. Research indicates that women who metabolize more of their estrogen at 2OH are likely to have a lower risk of breast cancer (Taioli et al., 2010).

PHASE 2 BIOTRANSFORMATION: In the second step of estrogen biotransformation, these active estrogen metabolites are hooked up with a chemical group that "chaperones" them safely from the body. The two major reactions in this step are methylation and glucuronidation. Supporting these two pathways is a key way we can improve the body's handling of estrogen and hormone-like chemicals. Interestingly, these reactions can be "undone" in the large intestine by unfriendly gut bacteria and estrogens released back into circulation.

Many different chemicals besides estrogen undergo biotransformation in the liver and each takes a specific path. Glucuronidation is the primary reaction for steroidal hormones, phenols, and benzoic acid. Other key reactions include glutathione conjugation of highly reactive molecules to form mercapturates (molecules that "capture" harmful substances and enable their excretion) and methylation.

BALANCING PHASE 1 AND PHASE 2 PROCESSES: The balance between Phase 1 and Phase 2 detoxification reactions is very important. Phase 1 reactions, as you recall, transform a substance from fat-loving to water-soluble. While now water soluble, the products of Phase 1 are often highly reactive. If the reactions from the first phase out-pace the rate of the second phase we can end up with more toxic substances circulating in the body.

The Power of Diet

Now that we have a sense of different kinds of chemicals that can be present in our bodies, food supply, and environment, we can take a look at what we call the power of diet and discuss steps we can take to manage a) limit our exposure and b) support our liver's detoxification efforts.

Dietary Practices That Support Our Body's Detoxification Processes

- Maintain a healthy body weight. As discussed in Chapter 2, our fat tissues can be a major contributor to estrogen levels in the body and can also serve as a "storage depot" for fat-soluble hormones and toxic chemicals.
- Follow the concrete steps in the last section to *limit exposure* to endocrine-mimicking chemicals like BPA, POPs, heavy metals, and phthalates.
- Eat organically raised fruits, vegetables, and animal products.
- Avoid sources of heavy metals, including exhaust fumes and fish.
- Certain foods can support the processes of Phase 1 and Phase 2 biotransformation. You've heard that eating your fruits and veggies is good for you … now here's another reason why!
- Protein includes good sources of sulfur-containing amino acids, cysteine, and methionine. The amino-acid building blocks of protein are essential for all liver enzymes, including the intercellular biggie: glutathione. Eating lean, bioavailable sources of protein from both vegetable and animal sources will support the body's ability to get rid of toxins.
- FIBER AND LIGNANS can bind free estrogen in the GI tract and promote excretion as feces. In addition, dietary fiber supports the health of beneficial gut bacteria and discourages overgrowth of bacteria that can re-digest estrogen and other toxic metabolites destined for excretion.
- INDOLE-3-CARBONYL, found in cruciferous vegetables like broccoli, cauliflower, and cabbage, has been shown to promote the 2OH pathway of estrogen metabolism.
- B-VITAMINS found in whole, unprocessed foods are usually present wherever you see an enzymatic reaction.

Another Plug for Diet: Epigenetics

At the 2010 American Society for Reproductive Medicine conference in Denver, the message from the experts studying the impact of environmental toxins on fertility was one of hope, with a focus on the emerging field of epigenetics—and a solution that may prove as simple as green leafy vegetables.

In simple terms, epigenetics is the study of how lifestyle factors like stress and diet can impact the way our inherited genetic makeup (our DNA) plays out without altering the genetic material itself. By now we are all fairly familiar with the term *genome,* which refers to the DNA strands that hold the blueprint for life. DNA is made up of sequences of nucleic acids (genes) that contain the "recipe" for all components and processes of cells. For a long time, scientists believed our DNA was the key determinant of our physical characteristics, including our risk for disease. But now the plot has thickened. Scientists have recently identified a new layer in the world of genetics: the epigenome.

To imagine what the epigenome is, think about an assortment of seeds that are dormant in a patch of earth, each with the potential to grow. Some of the seeds are beautiful wildflowers, others are weeds. The combination of sun, nutrients, temperature, and soil quality all determine whether the seeds grow or remain latent. The epigenome is analogous to a set of *conditions*—such as sunshine, adequate water, or frost—that either activate or deactivate DNA "seeds," or genes. Key players in the epigenome include proteins called *histones,* around which the strands of our DNA are wrapped, and special chemical groups, *methyl groups*, that act like "switches" that turn genes off and on. Changes to the shape of the histones or modifications to these chemical switches modify which genes are active and which remain dormant—all without any change to our inherited DNA code.

So what does any of this have to do with fertility? Well, one chemical in particular is receiving a great deal of attention for its association with infertility and negative birth outcomes. This chemical, mentioned above in our list of endocrine disruptors, is bisphenol-A (BPA).

Recently a team of researchers from Duke University identified the exact mechanism by which BPA affects female fertility. It turns out that HOXA10, a specific gene responsible for normal uterine development in mice and humans was chemically modified in the female offspring of pregnant mice treated with BPA. In particular, these offspring were found to have missing methyl groups in the HOXA10 gene. Females born to mice exposed to BPA had uterine tissue that was hypersensitive to estrogen and likely to be out of sync with the needs of developing embryos. As a result of this modification, the researchers said, these mice would ovulate/conceive normally but would be predisposed to having difficulty in *staying* pregnant.

The next step in this exploration was fascinating and has far-reaching implications for the potential treatment and prevention of infertility due to environmental exposure. After noting that BPA seemed to affect HOXA10 methylation of the female mice pups in utero, the researchers turned to nutrition for a potential solution. Familiar dietary compounds including folic acid, B vitamins, and s-Adenosyl methionine are known to be key components in our body's methyl-making pathways. So what if increasing amounts of methyl-donating nutrients in the diet could mitigate the impact of BPA? In a followup study, the Duke University team did just that. The findings were exciting. Supplementing the diets of BPA-treated mice with the methyl-donor folate or a phytoestrogen found in soy erased the effects of BPA in their female offspring. (Dolinoy et al. 2007)

While these findings may seem to be more relevant to pregnant women who are concerned about passing BPA-related problems on to their daughters, there are also grounds for believing that dietary intervention might provide protection against the negative impact of BPA in women who are currently trying to conceive. In fact, researchers in other areas of study where epigenetics are in play, such as in colorectal cancer and mental illness, are looking at dietary modification and folate supplementation as a novel treatment and/or prevention of these diseases in adults.

News that the environment is impairing our fertility is very discouraging, but this research offers a welcome glimmer of hope for many women who are trying to conceive. Taking steps to avoid toxic exposure is great—but many of the offending chemicals are found almost everywhere. Eating ample amounts of nutrients that support DNA methylation is an extra step we can take to empower ourselves and potentially deter negative effects from the environment.

Throughout this book we discuss the importance of eating ample amounts of fruits and vegetables as part of a fertility-friendly diet. Any woman who is trying to conceive should also be taking a prenatal vitamin that provides generous amounts of folate to guard against neural tube problems in the developing embryo.

But folate from prenatal supplements is not enough. Studies show that folate from food sources provide greater benefits than those from supplementation. In addition to good dietary intake, women should be aware of certain factors that can impair folate levels, including alcohol intake, smoking, conditions that challenge the intestinal mucosa (such as celiac disease), and congenital deficiencies in the enzymes necessary for folate metabolism.

The following are key nutrients that support the body's methylation processes and the foods where they are found:

- **FOLIC ACID**: Green leafy vegetables (romaine lettuce, spinach, endive, kale), sunflower seeds, liver
- **VITAMIN B12**: Meat, liver, shellfish, milk
- **VITAMIN B6**: Whole grains, vegetables, nuts, meat
- **CHOLINE**: Egg yolks, soy products, cooked meats
- **METHIONINE**: Sesame seeds, cottage cheese, Brazil nuts, fish, peppers, spinach

Breath, Yoga, And Fitness

THE PATHOPHYSIOLOGY OF STRESS

Scientists define stress as a physiological response to undesired emotional or physical situations. The initial physiological response to stress is an activation of the sympathetic nervous system that leads to a "fight-or-flight response," a series of rapid physical changes in the nervous system that readies the body for either escape or self-defense when a threat is detected.

In our previous book, *Fully Fertile*, we describe the stress response as the "Big Brown Bear Effect." While kind of silly, we still like this image of our great-great-great-great-grandmother (let's call her Gigi for short) hunting berries in the woods and looking up to find herself face to face with a cave bear. The moment Gigi looks up into that snarling face dripping with drool, her body kicks into survival mode—she must either fight or run. The hypothalamus, a tiny gland in the most primitive part of Gigi's already well-developed brain, sets off an alarm that causes a series of biological changes:

- The "stress hormones" adrenaline and cortisol are released by the adrenal glands, which are in charge of managing stress in the body. Adrenaline serves to focus the brain and stimulate cardiovascular action (increase heart rate and blood pressure), while cortisol works to release fuel to the muscles and increase the availability of substances necessary for tissue repair.
- Cortisol also works to down-regulate nonessential body function, including digestion and reproduction, and helps to shunt blood away from internal organs to the skeletal muscles.
- This short-term response is part of the sympathetic nervous system (SNS).

For Gigi, these are excellent changes. She is able to turn tail and run from the Big Brown Bear and return to the cave to share her hair-raising tale with the tribe. As Gigi sits by the fire and spins the tale, danger recedes and the levels of stress hormones in her blood return to normal.

But there's one more thing. You may know that the hypothalamus, the little almond-sized gland in Gigi's brain that started all this stress stuff, is located in a very ancient part of the human brain that is similar to animals, birds, and even reptiles. It is the part of our brain that recognizes danger. Gigi's human brain, however, has evolved a new self-awareness that is deeper than that of other animals. After the bear incident, Gigi may be a bit more nervous when she's out collecting berries. She may imagine or replay the event in her head. She may share her story with others, warning them to be careful. In essence, Gigi has the ability to know that she has experienced stress. Her neocortex, or higher brain, allows her to remember and, very importantly, to analyze her stressors.

In modern life, few of us will ever—knock on wood—experience the kind of physical danger that was part of Gigi's life. But although bears are not quite the threat they used to be our brains have found other things that seem to threaten our safety and happiness. Our Big Brown Bear is no longer just the furry kind; it's our smartphone, our commute, our mortgage, job stress, unemployment, and our complicated family relationships. It's infertility, fear of illness, and death.

When stress becomes chronic, it can play havoc with our health and well-being. Unlike adrenaline, cortisol levels take several days to return to normal. If stressful events follow in quick succession, as they often do in our "plugged-in" world, cortisol levels remain elevated almost continuously. In fact, cortisol—a hormone that is a vital part of the human survival strategy—can become one of the most toxic substances in our environment.

The effects of chronic stress are well documented. They include decreased cognitive acuity, changes in blood sugar regulation, decreased thyroid activity, impaired reproductive function, poor digestion, disruption of the immune system, and increased systemic inflammation.

A major part of the Cleanse Lifestyle involves learning to understand the source of stress in our lives and becoming skillful in handling stressful events and patterns of stress that have become imprinted in our minds and bodies. We will learn to elicit what Herbert Benson, MD, in his book of the same name, called *The Relaxation Response* (HarperTorch, August 1, 1976) which moves the body and mind from a state of "fight or flight" to one that allows for rest and repair. By the time you are finished with this section, you should have a better understanding of how certain techniques like deep breathing, yoga and exercise can each be used as physical strategies for coping with stress and eliciting the relaxation response. First, let's take a closer look at the physiology of the relaxation response.

UNDERSTANDING THE RELAXATION RESPONSE

Most of us are on intimate terms with the Stress Response (when the sympathetic nervous system is triggered) and its stomach- churning, heart-palpitating effects, but we're less familiar with the opposite state: the relaxation response (when the parasympathetic nervous system is engaged). During the relaxation response, the feeling in the body is one of "rest, digest, and nest." Heart palpitations and butterflies give way to a state where the body physiologically is in neutral, relaxed, and able to complete digestion and repair itself. You may notice that your tummy gurgles and rumbles and your heart and breathing rates slow. These two responses are closely related, and their prehistoric origins provide essential clues about how to stop stress in its tracks.

Meet the limbic system. This is the area of the human brain located around and within the brain stem. It is the oldest part of the human brain; in fact, it's so ancient it's often referred to as our "lizard brain," because its basic survival responses are similar in nature to those in the brains of primitive animals such as lizards and birds that preceded humans on the evolutionary ladder. The lizard brain (marginally better than bird-brain, right?) has three main organ "players":

THE HYPOTHALAMUS is concerned with maintaining the status quo in the body and regulates basic physical needs in the body, such as hunger, thirst, and sex drive. The hypothalamus regulates the autonomic nervous system, which controls both the Stress Response and the Relaxation Response, with input from the hippocampus and amygdala.

THE HIPPOCAMPUS takes short-term memory and sensory input and cements it into long-term memory.

THE AMYGDALA (there are two—one on the left and one on the right, about an inch behind the eyes and an inch in from the temples) is an almond-shaped organ that is involved with responding rapidly to stimuli that are perceived as a threat. When researchers have removed the amygdala of animals in experiments, those animals become indifferent to stimuli that might otherwise make them afraid, angry, or even sexually aroused.

So what does the limbic system have to do with the stress and/or relaxation responses? It's important to know that the three parts of the limbic system evolved to protect us. Any relaxation technique we use must work directly through these organs that work seamlessly and rapidly together to create a reaction to sensory input. This happens way before the big, fancy, human "reasoning" part of our mind can even figure out what's going on. Ever wonder why the smell of chocolate chip cookies makes your stomach growl? Why the sound of waves makes you want a pina colada and some romance? Why the smell of antiseptic can send you into a panic attack after a D&C? That's the limbic system. Thus, the relaxation techniques we propose in this book will often reach beyond the input of our "thinking" brain and look to sensory input, whether the afterglow of exercise, the sensations of stretching in yoga or the awareness of the breath to elicit our rest, digest and nest response. In the third section of this book we will even propose a relaxation ritual that uses the senses (sight, smell, etc.) to directly impact the limbic system.

You will also see this theme resurface in the second section of the book where we talk about cleansing the mind. This is a key concept and worth repeating: the stress response evolved before our fancy thinking brains. In many ways this short-circuiting of the thinking brain by returning to the sensory input of the current moment is the key to cleansing body and mind. For now, let's turn our attention to three powerful practices that help bring about the relaxation response in the body: The Breath, Yoga and Physical Exercise.

TECHNIQUE NO. 1: THE BREATH

It's very easy to eye-roll when someone tells you that deep breathing is an important cleansing technique. It sounds a) too simple to be true, and b) in the fertility arena this advice edges dangerously close to those polarizing words "just relax." Yet, there are strong scientifically acknowledged reasons why breathing may be an important catalyst in the fertility process.

Essentially, scientists have determined that humans have two basic breathing patterns. The first is "thoracic-dominant ventilation," which is typically characterized by a rapid, irregular breathing rate and a low tidal volume (amount of air that is exchanged in a given cycle of breath). In the thoracic pattern, the abdominal muscles are rigid (think suck in your gut!) and the shoulders and chest muscles tend to be tense. When you watch someone use thoracic breathing, you can often even see their shoulders rise and fall with the breath.

The second breathing pattern, "abdominal-diaphragmatic ventilation," a.k.a. "the belly breath," has a slow, rhythmic respiration rate and a relatively large tidal volume. In the abdominal pattern, the abdominal muscles are relaxed, and the belly moves outward on the inhale and relaxes back in on the exhale. You will not see shoulders move when someone is breathing into their belly.

Each of these breathing patterns is associated with distinct physiological effects. The one we want to use to promote fertility is definitely the belly breath.

Slow, rhythmic abdominal breathing creates a rise in carbon dioxide (CO_2) in the lung arterioles and, consequently, the blood. This increased (but still normal) level of CO_2 induces vascular relaxation, promotes blood flow to the brain, increases the excretion of acidic metabolites through the kidneys, and increases the transfer of oxygen from hemoglobin to tissues. Thoracic breathing, on the other hand, works in the opposite manner, decreasing CO_2 levels and causing constriction of blood flow in the heart and brain and less oxygen transfer to the tissues. In addition, belly breathing stimulates the vagus nerve, which controls important body functions such as respiration and digestion and sends sensory information to the brain. We'll discuss this important cranial nerve in more detail in the next section.

Since good blood flow and tissue oxygenation is important for fertility, these vascular actions are important. Using the belly breath has also been shown to shift the hormonal milieu in the body from "fight or flight," to "rest, digest, and nest."

Abdominal breathing also works for fertility on a mechanical level. When we relax the belly and breathe into the abdomen, the large, strong diaphragm muscle contracts downward. This action promotes the circulation of lymph, resulting in improved clearance of metabolic waste. The movement also massages the liver, stomach, intestines, and reproductive organs and stretches the connective tissue that surrounds the heart. When we release a belly breath, the upward motion of the muscle promotes the venous return of blood to the heart. Thoracic breathing, which is rapid and shallow, does not confer these benefits.

Close your eyes right now and focus on your breath. Identify your breathing pattern. Are your shoulders, back, and neck rigid as you breathe? Is your belly moving? If you're not using belly breath, try this exercise:

1. Sit in a straight-backed chair with your feet flat on the floor, or lie down.
2. Place one hand on your belly.
3. Close your eyes and begin to breathe in and out through your nose.
4. Breathe deep into the abdomen, feeling your belly expand with the inhale.
5. As you exhale, feel the hand and the belly gently move back toward the spine.

Continue this breathing pattern for 5-10 minutes. It may be helpful to visualize a balloon behind the navel that you inflate with the in-breath, and empty with the out-breath. With practice, this will become your habitual breathing pattern and you will reap the fertility-benefits of relaxation, better circulation, and a serene mind.

Stress and PTSD

Detox. Cleanse. Purify. These are familiar holistic buzzwords. But the process of trying to conceive can leave behind physical, emotional, even spiritual debris. So we may ask: Is there a way to "rid" ourselves of this negative stuff? And how do we protect ourselves from collecting more? From a holistic perspective, good nutrition, yoga, and sleep are simple strategies for detoxifying the *physical* body. Similarly, the mind and spirit are also able to release negativity—if we give them permission to do so. But what about the second question? Is there a way of protecting ourselves from negative baggage? Can we somehow create a shield around ourselves that keeps the disappointment from "sticking" and ruining our positive outlook?

Dr. Roger Pitman, a researcher and physician at Harvard University, has shown that the stress hormone adrenaline—which stimulates our "fight-or-flight" response—also serves to cement memories of trauma. (Pitman et al. 2002) Adrenaline, says Pitman, acts directly on the amygdala region of the brain, the part of the primitive limbic system concerned with fear and memory. In this theory, the stronger the adrenaline reaction to an event, the stronger and more lasting are the resulting fear and aversion—and the *memory* of the event.

Dr. Pitman's research focused on patients suffering from post-traumatic stress disorder (PTSD), but it is no overstatement to say that the failed IVFs, miscarriages, and losses involved in fertility challenges are major stressors, accompanied by huge levels of stress hormones. It's inescapable!

Or is it? The Harvard research found that it is our *response* to stress, rather than the actual stressful event, that is most involved in creating residual problems in the individual. The disappointments and traumas of infertility are certainly painful in and of themselves, but what if we learned to modulate our response or change our attitudes?

In our opinion, the simple, inexpensive techniques of yoga—stretching, breathing and meditation—really do create a defense against the onslaught of the stress response, and potentially, associated traumatic stress. One of the fundamental teachings of yoga is to learn how to calm and relax the body and mind. Stretching releases the physical patterns of dis-ease created by past physical and emotional trauma. Deep, calming belly breath helps lower levels of stress hormones circulating in the body, making us less "reactive" to stressful circumstances. The yoga practice of learning to observe our thoughts helps us identify and control patterns of negativity that allow routine events to spiral wildly into "worst-case" scenarios in our heads.

Beth writes: speaking from personal experience, yoga breathing in moments of trauma is of enormous benefit. The mindfulness we practice "on the mat" jumps into action in moments of trauma, reminding us that no matter what is happening externally, we have an inner peace that is unshakable. I can remember specific moments in the journey—during and after my stillbirth, through my other miscarriages, during the few weeks that both my boys spent in the Neonate Intensive Care Unit—when I was able to remind myself that the world was bigger than the immediate trauma I was experiencing through the basic technique of yoga breathing.

TECHNIQUE NO. 2: THE CLEANSING PRACTICE OF YOGA

In our opinion, possibly more than any other form of physical activity, yoga is effective at promoting radiant health and protecting the body from the ravages of stress, the environment, and even age to some extent. Why is yoga so effective?

First, yoga works the physical body in many different ways—folding, arching, stretching, and compressing the tissues of the body, and as a result creating strength, flexibility, and cardiovascular stamina at the same time. Yoga also works on the level of the mind: as the body becomes calmer and healthier, space is created where we then have an opportunity to look at the contents and patterns of our thoughts. Finally, yoga introduces a whole new paradigm of health and well-being—what we refer to as the "subtle" or "energetic realm." In this realm the currency of health is called *prana,* or "life force."

Much as we have different physiological systems and circuitry in the body, such as the respiratory and nervous systems, yoga anatomy also has a network of systems. The circuitry that carries prana throughout the body is known in Sanskrit as the *chakras* (wheels) and the *nadi* (pipes). There are seven main chakras in the body which align vertically along the spinal column as energy centers associated with physical, emotional and spiritual characteristics. It might be helpful to define the nadis as a super highway infrastructure that carries pranic energy from the base station of the seven chakras to all other areas of the body. Nadis in yoga are the same as meridians in Traditional Chinese Medicine. When these tubes get kinked or blocked, the energy/prana/qi does not flow freely back and forth from the chakras into the body which can result in physical or emotional distress or even illness. We will touch more fully on the nadis and chakras at the end of this chapter and recommend that if you wish to incorporate work with the chakras into your practice you consult a skilled yoga therapist or Reiki Master. You will find that it is helpful to have a knowledgeable and grounded guide as you enter the more esoteric areas of your practice.

To understand the subtle effects of yoga poses like how they might benefit the chakra system, it is helpful to understand more about the system of hatha yoga we are discussing here, and the philosophical tenets upon which it is founded.

The word *hatha* is composed of two Sanskrit terms, *ha*, which means "sun," and *tha*, which means "moon." Ha refers to the solar nadi in the body and tha refers to the lunar nadi in the body. Both of these tubes start on opposite sides of the spine and intertwine like vertical sine curves along the spine (think medical caduceus). They intersect at seven different locations along the spine and it is believed that these are the locations of the chakras. By combining the heat of the sun nadi (ha) with the cooling nature of the moon nadi (tha) a forceful energy is created. Thus, when read together, the word hatha means "powerful" in Sanskrit. The word yoga means "to yolk" or to bring together in equal parts. Hatha yoga, then, by definition is the power resulting when the energy of the sun is brought together with the energy of the moon in perfect balance. In other words, hatha yoga is a powerful purification process that is meant to bring opposing energies of the body into balance. This is largely done through physical stimulation of the chakras which is meant to unplug any kinks in the nadi system and allow prana to freely flow throughout the body. On a physical level the poses strengthen and purify body tissues. On a subtle level, these poses create a union of opposites (sun and moon, masculine and feminine, conscious and unconscious) that moves the practitioner into a higher state of awareness.

Exercise 1: Chakra Stimulating Sequence

Begin on your mat, on hands and knees, and take a moment to mindfully place your hands beneath your shoulders and align your knees under your hips. With an inhale, tip your tail bone skyward, releasing the ribs and belly downward and reach your collar bones and heart forward into Table Pose. Exhale, round your spine, take your seat to your heels and your head to the floor in Child's Pose. Now, inhale and come back to Table Pose. Then, with an exhale, lift the tail gently again and curl your toes under and press slowly into Downward-Facing Dog Pose. Let your head hang freely and begin to ease your heels toward the ground, gently straightening your legs. Come back down to Table Pose and repeat this series a few more times until you feel ready to rest for five full meditative minutes in Child's Pose.

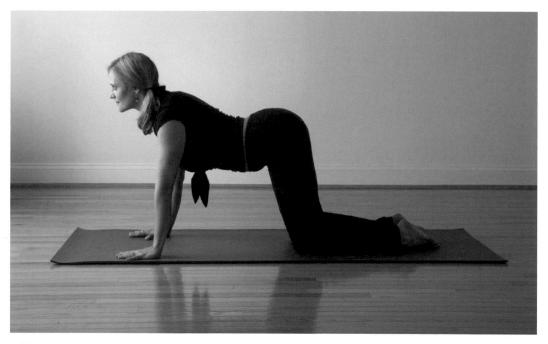

Table Pose

At first the experience in the sequence of yoga poses here is wholly physical—the muscles of the back, hamstrings, and calves stretch and the shoulders may quiver from bearing the weight of the body. As gravity pulls the head away from the spine, you may feel a lengthening, or feeling of "traction," in the spine. The mind registers these physical sensations as any number of things—delicious release, a frightening shift in equilibrium, or an uncomfortable stretch. Yet, as you continue to hold the pose and breathe into it a stillness arises within—a stillness in which you find you are able to observe the body's sensations and your mind's response to them. Finally, the body is flooded with new information and awareness about the body and mind processes related to this yoga experience.

The three distinct steps described in the exercise above—experiencing the physical sensation and the "mechanical work" of the pose, witnessing the mind's reaction to sensation, and remaining in "witness consciousness" while holding the pose—are the processes by which yoga can detoxify and heal our body. Together, they create *tapas,* the Sanskrit word in yoga for a purifying heat or energy. Tapas does not refer merely to physical heat; it also refers to the light of awareness that is kindled when we practice yoga poses mindfully. This cultivation of witnessing awareness, in our opinion, is the penultimate cleansing power of yoga.

Yoga Mechanics: The Physical Realm

Because we are trained to take a body-centric view of health, it's easiest to understand the cleansing nature of yoga on the physical level. Yoga poses have several distinct mechanical actions: they stretch, strengthen, fold, extend, twist, and invert. Each of these actions is associated with an energetic quality as well as a physical/mechanical effect. When we stretch we create space, and when we strengthen we create stability. We can think of the twisting as wringing out muscles and organs, much as we wring out a wet wash cloth. Postures that invert the body (i.e., position us where our head is beneath our heart) play with the laws of gravity to stimulate the body's nervous and cardiovascular systems.

Understanding a bit about the mechanics of a pose is the first step in understanding how yoga can help us cleanse. Once we understand the mechanics of the poses, we can discuss the energetic effects—how these poses affect the energy systems of our body: the nadis and the chakras.

STRETCHING

Stretching is perhaps the most obvious mechanical action of the yoga pose. But actually understanding what happens when we stretch allows us to be more fully present with the experience. To create movement, the fibers of our skeletal muscles contract and move the complex system of levers and joints that make up our skeletal system. After muscle contraction, however, a muscle fiber does not always return to its fully relaxed length. When muscle tension is not completely released—as occurs in cases of frequent strenuous exercise, chronic poor posture, or sustained fight-or-flight mode, the muscles in the body may actually begin to shorten and the muscle fibers can become "disorganized." In addition, the connective tissue (fascia) that surrounds muscle fibers can also shorten and stiffen.

The net result of this shortening and stiffening situation is tight bundles of muscle and connective tissue that decrease joint mobility, restrict blood flow, and have a negative effect on posture. As you know, restricting blood flow is not optimal for fertility. The right kind of stretching, however, can reverse this process.

When we stretch a muscle, the initial action simply returns the muscle to its fully relaxed length. From a broader perspective, this is a powerful cleansing action. If we deepen the stretch once the muscle has returned to its original state, the surrounding fascia absorbs the stretch. As the fascia bundles are elongated farther, they in turn "hug" muscle fibers into better alignment for better contractile function in the future.

Stretching can also help to heal old injury. When a muscle is torn or strained, the body does not repair the rupture with new muscle. The repair is made with scar tissue that is brittle, fibrous, and inflexible. It binds to the soft tissue and shrinks, closing the tear. The shrinking action of the scar tissue can pull other surrounding tissues out of shape and actually impede blood flow to and through the area. The result is a repair that is weaker than the original tissue, and the surrounding tissues may also suffer.

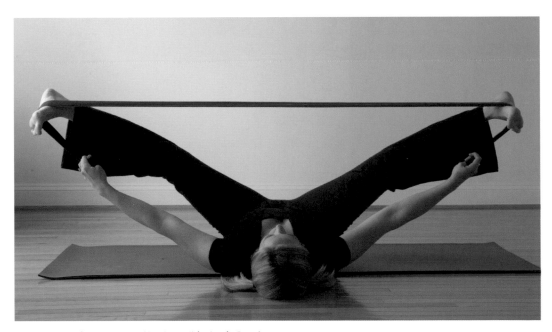

Supta Upavistha Konasana (Supine Wide Angle Pose)

Emotional factors can impact our skeletal system as well. In the face of shame, disappointment, and anger, it is common to contract emotionally and physically. We seek to protect ourselves from pain, so we avoid contact with people and situations that remind us of these negative emotions. The physical body can also contract in response to emotions. Grinding our teeth; tense muscles in the back, neck, shoulders, and abdomen; and tension headaches all result from emotional stress.

Energetically, the quality associated with stretching is one of creating space. Regular stretching actually prevents our connective tissue from becoming stiff and inflexible. Stretching and massage can actually break down scar tissue and improve blood flow to areas of past injury. When we stretch and move with our yoga practice, we are literally rehabilitating our muscular-skeletal system, healing past injury, and keeping our muscles and their surrounding connective tissue flexible.

Key fertility mantra words to chant while stretching:
"Flexible." "Fluid."

STRENGTH (AND STABILITY)

Many new yoga practitioners are shocked at how much work yoga can be. This is because yoga, in addition to being a stretching exercise, is equally concerned with creating strength and stability in the body. We see how necessary this is with elderly people, who tend to frequently lose their balance and fall, breaking bones easily.

On a structural level, strength is important because any work to increase the flexibility of our joints could ultimately lead to injury due to over-mobility. There are even a handful of people (we affectionately call them "gumbies") who are super bendy and fall into the most difficult yoga poses with ease. Unfortunately it is often the gumby types who are injured through their yoga practice. Loose joints allow them to bend and fold beyond safe limits. The strength/flexibility relationship is another example of the union of opposites embedded in the hatha yoga system. Without stability flexibility is useless, and vice versa.

Poses that encourage strength, such as standing poses, also create a simulated stress environment. As we move into the second phase of practice, witnessing the mind's reaction to the physical action, it's very clear that messages like "ugh, this is too hard," and "how long is my teacher going to make us hold this pose?" are stress messages from the brain. Our breath rate and heart rate may even increase in response to both these physical and mental responses. Relaxation after a strenuous pose is welcome and beneficial. By taking our stress system through its entire cycle—arousal to rest—we optimize its function.

Sthira sukham asanam: "The posture is stable and comfortable"

This is a famous phrase from the ancient text *The Yoga Sutras of Patanjali* and sums up the importance of finding a balance between effort and ease (the sun and the moon) in all aspects of life. Our hatha yoga practice allows us to carefully consider this recommendation in action as we find the right mixture of strength and stretch in each pose. When we practice yoga, we should always look to find that middle ground where we feel safe and stable yet are pushing ourselves—just a bit—to the outermost limits of our comfort zone. This is the place we want to be in our yoga place, that very fine line between comfort and discomfort.

Key fertility mantra words to chant during strengthening poses:

"Warrior"

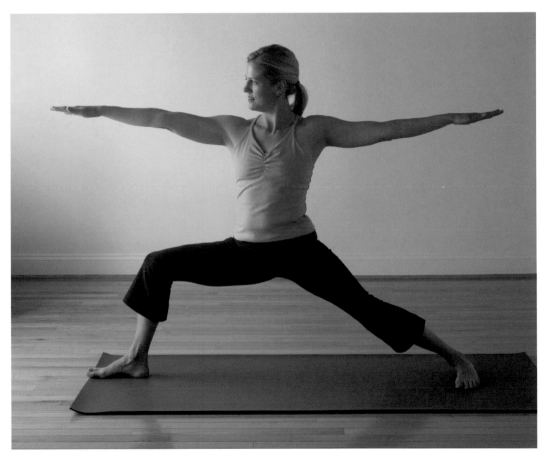

Virabhadrasana (Warrior Two Pose)

FORWARD FOLDS AND BACKBENDS

Like stretching and strengthening, the actions of folding forward and bending backward can be viewed as opposites, with different physiological and energetic effects. Forward folds are calming. They release tight musculature in the hamstrings, hips, back, and neck. Folding decreases heart rate and blood pressure and stimulates digestion. Backbending, on the other hand, strengthens and creates flexibility in the front side of the body. Backbends are the "espresso" of yoga—big energy and strong stimulation.

On an energetic level, backbends both stretch the back body—associated in yoga physiology with past and unconscious patterns—and stimulate the first, second, and third chakras, which are associated with survival, creativity, and personal power, respectively. Backbending is about opening the heart and letting go of fear, so that we can reach beyond ourselves and engage fully in the activities of the higher chakras: love and compassion, authentic expression, and wisdom.

A good yoga teacher will take you through a series of postures consisting of both forward folding and backbends, in order to allow the body to feel physically and energetically balanced. If you've ever done a yoga practice consisting primarily of backbends, you may have left feeling agitated, nervous, or "wired." Similarly, while a class filled with all forward bends can be

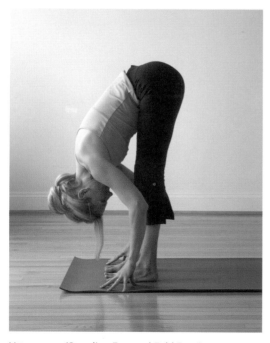

Uttanasana (Standing Forward Fold Pose)

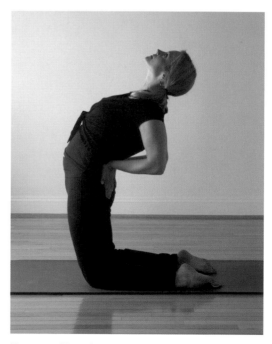

Ustrasana (Camel Pose)

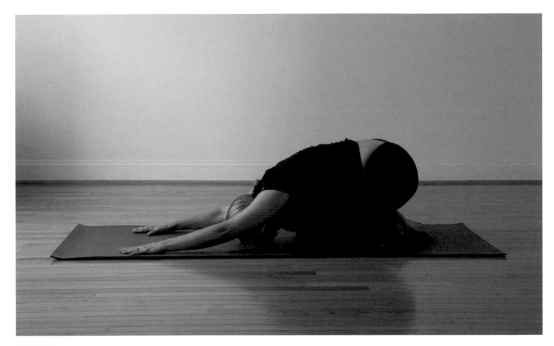

Child's Pose

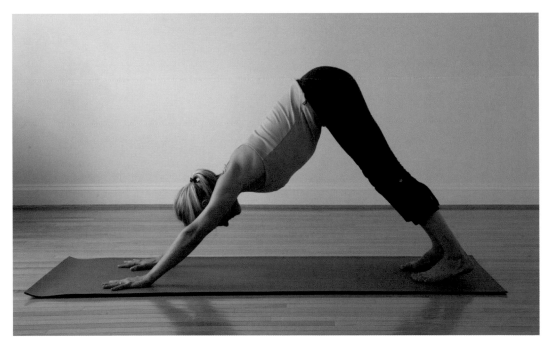

Downward-Facing Dog Pose

soothing, and even slow down the central nervous system, it can also create a feeling of sluggishness. As we've mentioned before, everything in life, including your yoga practice, should be balanced between opposite extremes.

Key fertility mantra words to chant during forward folds and backbends:

Forward Folds: "Calm"

Backbends: "Open"

TWISTING

The mechanical action of twisting poses has been described as "squeeze and soak." The posture first compresses muscles and organs, forcing out blood and fluid filled with metabolic waste. When the pose is released, fresh blood flows in to oxygenate and nourish the tissues. Twists also serve to improve our posture and the health of our spine. When we twist it is imperative that we keep a straight spine, with the crown of the head directly in line with the sacrum.

We must also respect that the three main parts of our spine differ in their ability to rotate. The cervical spine (in the neck) has the most mobility. The thoracic spine, which is connected to our ribcage, is more limited. And the lumbar spine, which is integrated into the sacrum and

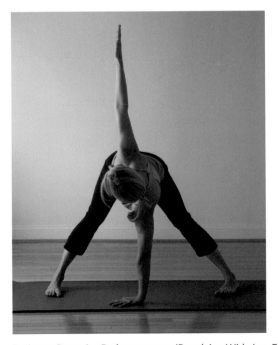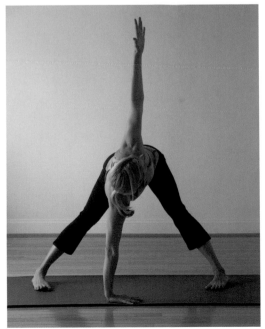

Parivrtta Prasarita Padottanasana (Revolving Wide Leg Forward Fold Pose)

pelvic bones, has limited mobility. Twists serve to tone and stretch a group of muscles that are considered "postural" muscles in the low back and abdomen. Postural muscles can be thought of as the "strong silent type"—they provide stability rather than flash. Postural muscles include the erector spinae, quadratus lumborum, and abdominal obliques. Challenging these muscles to contract and move helps to stimulate blood flow into these areas that tend to be more static—a great thing for both detoxification and fertility.

On an energetic level, twisting poses signify a sort of "out with the old, in with the new." Because they create a spiral, they cause us to be aware of where we have been and where we are going simultaneously. Even though the primary movement of the twist is revolution around the spine, as we continue to practice and explore twists we also recognize they help us to lengthen and maintain the integrity of the spine (our center line). This upward movement is symbolic of evolution. We're not just talking about change; we're talking about change for the better.

Key fertility mantra words to chant during twists:
"Change"

BALANCE POSES

Most fundamental balance postures in yoga require standing on one foot, so we will focus on these poses rather than arm balances for the purposes of your fertility cleanse. A well-grounded foot is what creates a steady and strong foundation for the pose. Most often, the inner arch of the foot feels slightly lifted and light, while the base of the big toe and the inner heel remain firmly grounded.

The muscle that grounds the big toe, the peroneus longus, lies along the outer calf. Its tendon crosses the outer ankle and then the sole of the foot before attaching to the bottom of the bones that form the innermost part of the arch; when it's engaged, you sense a sort of firmness in the outer calf and you will feel as though the mound of the big toe is pressing downward into the earth. The tibialis anterior, one of the main muscles that supports the arch, lies along the outer surface of the shinbone on the front of the lower leg. Ideally, you should be able to sense a balance between the tibialis anterior lifting the arch and the peroneus longus grounding the base of the big toe.

The balancing action of the foot and lower leg is very important. True beginners may want to simply play with the idea of lifting one foot and balancing on the other without feeling tippy. Too much weight in either the toe or the heel can make you feel off kilter. Once you've mastered the toe and lower leg, move your attention to your pelvis, which transfers weight from your torso to your standing leg. If the pelvis twists, turns, or leans to one side, it will throw off the entire pose. It is important for the pelvis to align directly over the standing leg. The hips also play an important role in holding the pelvis stable and, if you dig your thumb

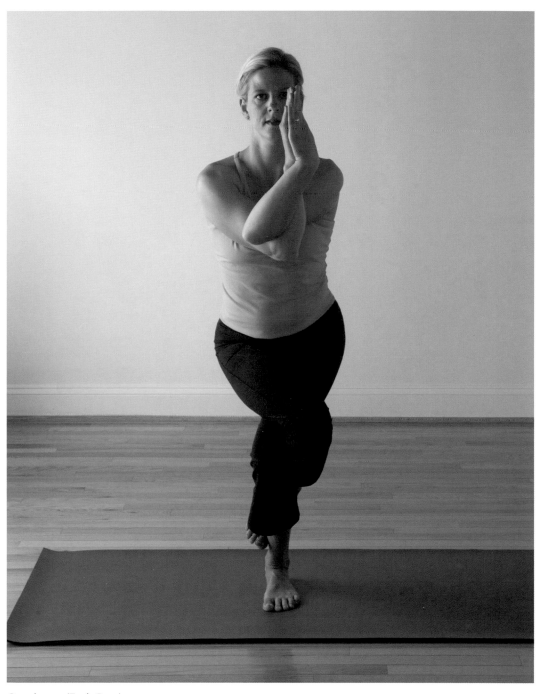

Garudasana (Eagle Pose)

into them while balancing, you may be able to feel them contract. In time, you will come to admire your balance postures for the symphony of muscles and body parts that must work together to make standing on one leg possible. Often, for yoga novices, the actions involved in balance poses are so radically different that just *thinking* about the mechanics of balance poses can develop new neurological pathways.

On an energetic level, balance poses help train our minds to be focused and present in the moment. We challenge anyone to think about their "to do" list while balancing on one foot. This sort of extreme focus and centering will spill over into other areas of your life beyond the yoga mat. You may find you are better able to concentrate at work, be present with your loved ones, or savor beautiful experiences happening right now.

Key fertility mantra words to chant during balance postures:

"Here"

INVERSIONS

It's easy to understand inversions by thinking of anything that is upside down or in an opposite position. By definition, however, an inversion in yoga is any posture where the head is lower than the heart (mild inversions) or the feet are higher than the heart (full inversions). There is much debate as to whether inversions should be practiced during a menstrual cycle or during certain phases of pregnancy, and should be approached with caution by people with low blood pressure. Ancient yogic tradition states the inversions should not be practiced when a woman is menstruating, nor during certain phases of pregnancy. Many yoga teachers scoff at this notion, saying that these limitations must have been conjured up by men because there is no biological reason why a woman can't invert throughout her menstrual cycle and/or pregnancy.

While this issue can be debated at length, Pulling Down the Moon takes the side of the ancients. It is our belief that during a menstrual cycle, nothing should be done that would reverse the flow of blood from out of the uterus. It is an important part of our monthly uterine cleanse and, at the same time, allows an energetic clearing from inside the body, down and out. In traditional Chinese medicine (TCM), it is believed that stagnating blood left in the uterus can lead to endometriosis, painful menses, and even severe clotting.

When it comes to the issues of doing inversions during pregnancy, Pulling Down the Moon does believe that inversions done in the last trimester to turn a breach pregnancy can be useful if taught by a yoga instructor who is certified and experienced in prenatal yoga. Pulling Down the Moon does not recommend inversions at other times during the pregnancy. Certain inverted postures are fine to perform during menstruation and pregnancy, such as Legs Up the Wall Pose and Downward-Facing Dog Pose (considered by some to be an inversion).

Inversions have a great many benefits for fertility, such as reversing the flow of blood from the legs into the areas of the head and reproductive organs. Inversions can also aid in digestion, lymphatic drainage, and increasing blood flow to the heart.

On an energetic level, inversions turn our world upside down. They often help us see things from a different perspective—you know, up is down and down is up. They can increase our focus, aid our sleep, and help us to think more clearly. Perhaps most importantly, doing inversions can help create a great sense of accomplishment within us. Being upside down and balancing at the same time, as required in handstands, requires not only balance and strength but a tremendous amount of courage in trusting that we will be okay and not topple over.

Key fertility mantra words to chant during inversion postures:

"Fearlessness"

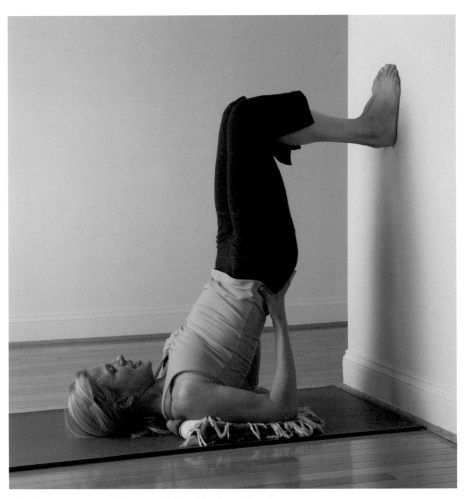

Salamba Sarvangasana (Supported Shoulder Stand Pose)

Yoga and Stress Reduction Benefits

A new study examining the potential stress-reduction benefits of hatha yoga practice (Kiecolt-Glaser et al, 2010) compared the inflammatory and endocrine responses of healthy women to a restorative hatha yoga session and to control activity. Half of the 50 subjects were "expert yoginis" (women with a regular yoga practice) and half were yoga novices. Prior to each intervention session, the women were subjected to stress challenges in order to gauge the extent that yoga speeds recovery from stress. The results of the study were very interesting.

1. The yoga session boosted mood compared to the control activities, but no change was found in subjects' response to stress before and after yoga or any of the control sessions.
2. However, in response to the stress events, the novices, who were not different in age or other variables from the experts, had measured levels of C-reactive protein levels (a marker of inflammation) that were 4.75 times higher than the yoga experts. The researchers concluded that a regular yoga practice lowers the impact of stressful events.

These findings are extremely relevant for women struggling with infertility. Stress is an inflammatory condition, and inflammation is implicated in many infertility diagnoses, including PCOS, endometriosis, miscarriage, and potentially even poor egg and sperm quality.

The take-home from this research is that yoga may do more for a woman who is trying to conceive than reduce her anxiety levels and improve her mood. Regular yoga practice may actually improve her physiological response to stress events and protect her body from the negative effects of chronic inflammation.

Yoga Energetics: The Subtle Realm

MORE ON THE UNION OF OPPOSITES

At the beginning of this chapter when we defined *hatha yoga* and discussed its cleansing power, we mentioned the union of opposites at work and how they present themselves on physical, energetic, and spiritual levels. Physically, hatha yoga postures can be either asymmetrical or symmetrical. If a pose is asymmetrical, it is generally practiced on both on sides. In practicing an asymmetrical pose, the student may notice and address differences in strength, coordination, and flexibility on opposite sides of the body. Practicing a symmetrical pose can be deeply calming, as we physically experience the union of opposites. Energetically, hatha yoga works to balance feminine and masculine energy. Analogous to the forces of yin and yang that inform Traditional Chinese Medicine (TCM), feminine energy (yin) is emotional, nurturing, and latent and is symbolized by the moon. Masculine energy (yang) is analytical, extroverted, and active and represented by the sun.

Hatha yoga poses can be lunar or solar in their essence. For instance, Warrior 1 Pose and Chair Pose are energetic poses that generate heat and energy in the body. Forward Folds and Supta Baddha Konasana are cooling poses that can release pent-up heat and energy from the body. Practiced in series, hatha yoga poses can be used to create a balanced energetic effect.

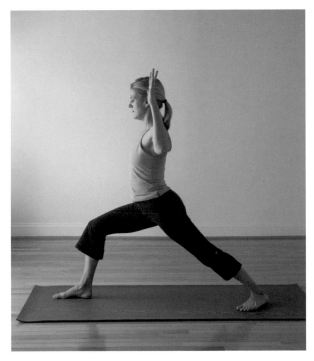

Modified Virabhadrasana I (Modified Warrior I)

Utkatasana (Chair Pose)

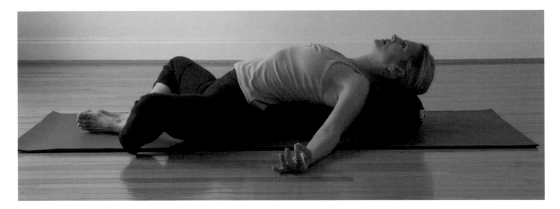

Supta Baddha Konasana (Supine Cobbler's Pose)

THE IDA, PINGALA, AND SUSHUMNA NADIS

By now you have come to understand that when we speak of energy in yoga we are referring to *prana*, the life force. Prana is like electricity: it exists in the natural world as the raw energy of life—as electricity is present in lightning, static, and friction. Like electricity, prana can be channeled through the circuitry of the *nadis* to conduct life force throughout the body.

There are three main nadis that originate at the base of our spine: the *pingala*, the *ida* and the *sushumna*. You are already familiar with two of these nadis, the pingala which we previously referred to as the "sun channel" and the ida which we formerly called the "moon channel." The central channel, called the *sushumna nadi*, runs directly from the base of the spine to the crown of the head. The ultimate and life-long goal of yoga is to balance prana within the ida and pingala so that energy is guided up and down the sushumna. When this happens, the chakras become energized and the individual often experiences a state of euphoria (*Samadhi*), clear-mindedness, balance or a period of spiritual awakening. Often the feelings of euphoria last only a few seconds, minutes or hours. The practice is to achieve this state of grace with greater frequency and duration. Here's a quick reference to summarize the three main nadis in our energetic anatomy along with their corresponding attributes:

IDA: Originates at the base of the spine and moves left, then wraps around the sushumna as it spirals to the top of the head. It is associated with feminine energy, the moon (tha) and intuition.

PINGALA: Starts at the base of the spine and winds right, wraps around the sushumna like the ida, and is associated with sun (ha), masculine energy, and the power of reason.

SUSHUMNA: The center channel representing the balance of the ida and the pingala. It runs from the base of the spine to the crown of the head. It controls our spiritual evolution and is believed to connect this world with the next.

THE CHAKRAS

If the nadis are the roads along which life energy travels, chakras are the roundabouts that direct life force throughout the body. Chakras are thought to be junction points between body and that which is beyond body (mind, spirit, personal evolution). Ancient sages "saw" the chakras as a series of energy wheels (again *chakra* means "wheel") located along the axis of our spine. Each energy center is associated with a color and with a particular area of spiritual evolution. Interestingly, each chakra is also associated with an endocrine gland—the master glands that orchestrate physical and emotional health.

It is tempting to use the chakras as a diagnostic tool (e.g., infertility = second chakra issues). But as with everything else, these energy wheels work as part of a sort of electric circuitry in the body. Shorts, blockages, and overages in any one part can create hiccups in the entire system. It is not accurate to simply hone in on one chakra and think the entire system can be cured.

The seven chakras and their associated functions are as follows:

FIRST CHAKRA: Muladhara Chakra (Survival)
COLOR: Red
ENDOCRINE ASSOCIATION: Adrenals

The Muladhara Chakra is located at the very base of the spine and is also called the "root chakra." This energy center relates to our sense of safety, and the sense of "belonging" either to a family or larger group. When this chakra is open and conducting energy freely, we feel secure and are confident that our needs are being met. Blocks in the Muladhara Chakra bring anxiousness and worry. We can envision this chakra as connected to the earth and access the grounded energy of earth through it.

SECOND CHAKRA: Svadisthana Chakra (Creativity)
COLOR: Orange
ENDOCRINE ASSOCIATION: Ovaries/Testes

Ever wonder why the color of fertility is orange? You can thank the Svadisthana Chakra, or the "fertility" chakra. From this energy center flows our ability to create and to birth—literally, as in children—but also the ability to create and express different parts of our selves. When this chakra is open and conducting energy freely, we are connected to a vibrant energy that simply wants to create and to share. If this chakra is blocked, we may feel infertile, dry and brittle. We can envision this chakra as connected to a fountain of creative energy. Again, just because you might be experiencing infertility, it doesn't necessarily mean that you have something wrong with your second chakra.

THIRD CHAKRA: Manipura Chakra (Power)
COLOR: Yellow
ENDOCRINE ASSOCIATION: Pancreas

The Manipura Chakra is the seat of our personal power and sense of self-actualization. When this chakra is open and conducting energy freely, we feel confident and connect with our ability to achieve our goals. When blocked, we feel frustrated and ineffectual. We can envision this chakra as connected to the radiant energy of the sun, the power that helps things grow.

FOURTH CHAKRA: Anahata Chakra (Heart and Beauty)
COLOR: Green
ENDOCRINE ASSOCIATION: Thymus

The Anahata Chakra is also called the heart chakra because it is connected to love and compassion, emotions that resonate with our hearts. Unlike the first three chakras, which are concerned with self, the fourth chakra looks outward to others. When the Fourth Chakra is open, we feel a deep connection with others; when it is blocked, we can feel lonely and isolated. We can envision this chakra as connected to the radiant energy of love, compassion, and beauty.

FIFTH CHAKRA: Vishudda Chakra (Communication)
COLOR: Blue
ENDOCRINE ASSOCIATION: Thyroid

The fifth chakra is all about truth—our truth and authenticity and our ability to speak and share clearly and intelligently. When this chakra is blocked, we may not feel comfortable speaking, we may lie, or we may be easily misunderstood. We can envision this chakra as connected with the powerful energy of sound.

SIXTH CHAKRA: Ajna Chakra (Intuition)
COLOR: Purple
ENDOCRINE ASSOCIATION: Pituitary

Also known as the "third eye," the sixth chakra is the seat of our innate wisdom and intuition. When this chakra is clear and conducting energy freely we trust in the flow of life, feel confident about our choices and our insights. When blocked, we may find it hard to trust ourselves and others and may feel confused. We can envision this chakra as tapped into the power of intuition and clear seeing.

SEVENTH CHAKRA: Sahaswara Chakra (Divinity)
COLOR: White
ENDOCRINE ASSOCIATION: Hypothalamus

Also called the "crown chakra," the seventh chakra is our connection with our highest self. When this chakra is open, we are aware of our connection with greatness, with pure awareness, and with unfading joy. This chakra is thought to burst open when we acknowledge our own divine nature.

Starting a Yoga Practice

In the third section of the book you will find photos of the yoga practices that accompany this book and also serve as a companion practice for our first book *Fully Fertile*. That book is a tremendous resource for in-depth information about the use of yoga for fertility. It is our goal that you will use these practices as a jumping off point for your own exploration of hatha yoga. As always, please clear any exercise program with your physician before diving in.

TECHNIQUE NO. 4: FERTILITY-FRIENDLY FITNESS

What about other forms of exercise? Are they part of the Cleanse Lifestyle? Many women decide (or are told to) stop exercising when they are trying to conceive. This piece of bad advice, which likely arose from the association between very strenuous exercise and infertility, needs to be rectified immediately. Women who are trying to conceive should definitely exercise for many, many reasons. At Pulling Down the Moon, we use a sort of "decision tree" to help women find an exercise regimen that's right for them, asking the following questions:

1. HOW CLOSE ARE YOU TO YOUR IDEAL BODYWEIGHT?

As discussed earlier, body weight can play a major role in fertility, with some women being too lean for proper hormone function or too heavy, where excesses of estrogen-producing adipose tissue (fat) disrupts hormonal balance. For women who are close to their optimal weight, an exercise program should serve to reduce stress, develop/maintain strength, and keep the heart healthy. Women who need to *lose* weight should set goals to increase daily activity levels significantly through a program of low impact cardiovascular exercise, strength training, and stress-reduction activities such as yoga. If you're not sure about your ideal weight, a consultation with a nutritionist is a great place to start.

2. WHAT ROLE HAS EXERCISE PLAYED IN YOUR LIFE UP TO THIS POINT?

Some women have a less-than-healthy relationship with physical exercise. Some may hate it and struggle to fit it in to their day. Chronic under-exercise can make it hard to maintain a healthy body weight or may contribute to sluggishness and depression. On the flip side, there are those of us who train hard every day, use exercise to maintain an "ideal" body weight, or feel anxious when exercise is limited. Chronic over-exercise can raise levels of the stress hormone cortisol, as well as negatively affect the function of the hypothalamic-pituitary-ovarian axis (the hormonal system that governs reproductive function). Your relationship with exercise will dictate whether you need to slow down or speed up.

Once we know the answers to the questions above, we can begin to make recommendations. In general, a fertility-friendly exercise program should include cardiovascular exercise that is low-impact and low to medium intensity, which means keeping our heart rate under 60 percent of cardiac capacity. Strength training is also fabulous when you're trying to conceive, as it increases lean muscle mass and helps keep the body strong and shapely (although we need to be careful here—a body fat percentage of at least 22 percent is generally accepted as necessary for a regular menstrual cycle). In addition to looking good, lean mass increases metabolism and builds stronger bones.

Yoga is another must-try for those who are trying to conceive. As we explored in detail above, the yoga asanas increase strength, improve our flexibility, and help to balance our hormones. Yoga has been proven to reduce levels of cortisol, and in yoga physiology it's believed that specific yoga postures can be used to increase the flow of blood and life force (prana) to reproductive organs.

Exercise may also protect against oxidative stress. The word *aerobic* means "occurring in the presence of oxygen." During aerobic exercise, the body obviously consumes a great deal of oxygen, and as a result creates a significant amount of reactive oxygen species (ROS). While on the surface this may seem like a bad thing, it is not. In fact, the oxidative stress generated by physical exercise may actually train body tissues to produce more antioxidant enzymes and scavenge free radicals more efficiently (Fisher-Wellman et al., 2009).

Exercise confers other benefits for women who are trying to conceive. It can help us maintain a healthy body weight. Regular moderate-intensity aerobic exercise improves glucose transport from circulating blood sugar into the mitochondria, or energy powerhouses in the cells, thereby directly improving blood sugar regulation and energy.

Exercise can reduce stress and improve mood. This is a time for nurturing, fun activity. Take walks outside, ride a bike for pleasure and sight-seeing, and enjoy an energizing yoga practice. Exercise when you're trying to conceive should help you reduce stress, but should not leave you overly fatigued or sore. This is not the time to train for a marathon, shave a minute off your running speed, or "get ripped" working out with weights in the gym.

Cleansing the Mind

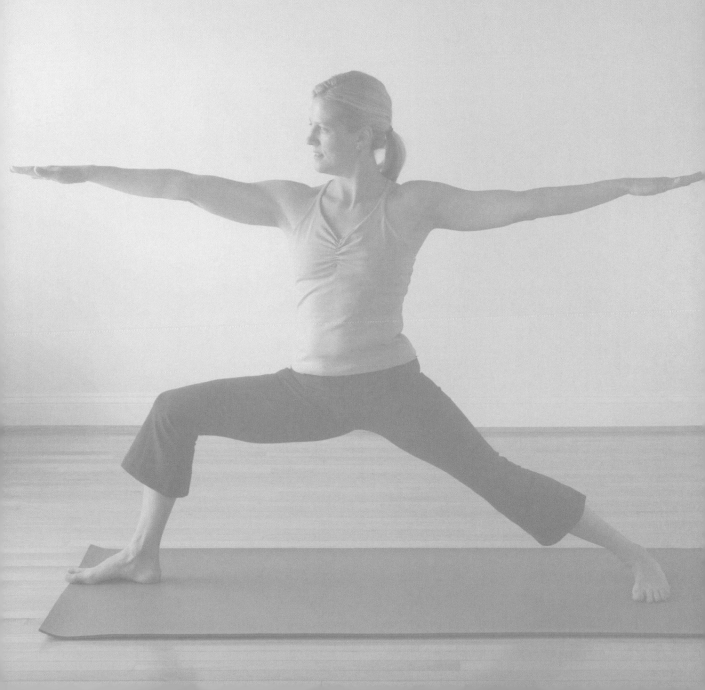

CHAPTER 5

Toxins of the Mind

Y ou have just completed the first section of the book, which offers an in-depth discussion about the ways in which your body and physical surroundings encounter toxins every day. We presented both a physiological and scientific approach to the detoxification process, including information about the ways in which the liver, kidneys, and skin help eliminate toxins. We can take steps to minimize our exposure to toxins, and practices we can adopt to help our bodies manage the toxic load. These include choosing to put only good things in our bodies and avoiding harmful chemicals.

We will be providing you with further "Detox Practices" and other support materials in the last section of the book. Now, though, we want to introduce a concept that some of you may find challenging. Perhaps the idea isn't so radical, but some of the practices and ideas we will introduce later in the section will be, so hold onto your hat.

Okay, here goes: Stress acts as a huge toxin in the body.

We're sure most of you are not surprised to hear that stress is toxic; more surprising, perhaps, is that you can actually use your mind to detox your body.

Like the chicken and the egg, it's difficult to know exactly which came first. Is it that the mind has a thought and we create stress around it? Or is it that we have stress and the mind creates a thought? We can ask this same question when it comes to the stress and infertility debate. Does stress cause infertility? Does infertility cause stress? Or are they so interrelated that both need to be addressed?

Let's start with the six-million-dollar question first: Does stress cause infertility?

THE STRESS AND INFERTILITY DEBATE

At Pulling Down the Moon fertility centers, we have found that many women believe stress is a major contributor to their infertility. In an attempt to be faithful to clinical evidence, and since we work with medical doctors at Pulling Down the Moon, we are always digging into the literature in an attempt to learn more about new studies, old studies, and anything in between that would help point the arrow in one direction or another: either stress causes infertility or it doesn't.

Let's start with the current standard medical view. The American Society of Reproductive Medicine (ASRM) publishes a patient fact sheet on its website that addresses the whole idea of stress and infertility. We are reprinting it here so you have a better understanding of how your doctor might perceive your stress in the mix of your medical fertility treatment. Encouragingly, medical doctors agree that a disciplined lifestyle can go a long way toward helping a woman manage the stress of infertility. Indeed, ASRM encourages women who wish to conceive to follow a good diet (e.g., eliminating stimulants such as caffeine) and to use stress-reduction techniques like meditation, yoga, and acupuncture.

PATIENT FACT SHEET
STRESS AND INFERTILITY

Published with permission of ASRM as it appears on ASRM.org

Stress can come from just about anything that you feel is threatening or harmful. A single event (or your worry about it) can produce stress. So can the little things that worry you all day long.

Acute stress, caused by a single event (or your fear of it), makes your heart beat faster and your blood pressure go up. You breathe harder, your hands get sweaty, and your skin feels cool and clammy. Chronic stress, which is when you are always stressed, can cause depression and changes in your sleep habits. It can also decrease your chances of fighting off common illnesses. Stress makes many body organs work harder than normal and increases the production of some important chemicals in your body, including hormones.

Is stress causing my infertility?
Probably not. Even though infertility is very stressful, there isn't any proof that stress causes infertility. In an occasional woman, having too much stress can change her hormone levels and therefore cause the time when she releases an egg to become delayed or not take place at all.

Is infertility causing my stress?
Maybe. Many women who are being treated for infertility have as much stress as women who have cancer or heart disease. Infertile couples experience stress each month: first they hope that the woman is pregnant; and if she is not, the couple has to deal with their disappointment.

Why is infertility stressful?

Most couples are used to planning their lives. They may believe that if they work hard at something, they can achieve it. So when it's hard to get pregnant, they feel as if they don't have control of their bodies or of their goal of becoming parents. With infertility, no matter how hard you work, it may not be possible to have a baby. Infertility tests and treatments can be physically, emotionally, and financially stressful. Infertility can cause a couple to grow apart, which increases stress levels. Couples may have many doctor appointments for infertility treatment, which can cause them to miss work or other activities.

What can I do to reduce my stress?

- Talk to your partner.
- Realize you're not alone. Talk to other people who have infertility, through individual or couple counseling, or support groups.
- Read books on infertility, which will show you that your feelings are normal and can help you deal with them.
- Learn stress reduction techniques such as meditation, yoga, or acupuncture.
- Avoid taking too much caffeine or other stimulants.
- Exercise regularly to release physical and emotional tension.
- Have a medical treatment plan with which both you and your partner are comfortable.
- Learn as much as you can about the cause of your infertility and the treatment options available.
- Find out as much as you can about your insurance coverage and make financial plans regarding your fertility treatments.

The Controversy Continues

At the time of writing, in 2011, a new study has been published by researcher Jacky Boivin (Boivin et al, 2011) showing that a woman's stress level does not impact the success rate of IVF. The research analyzed data from 14 studies measuring women's stress during IVF and found no correlation between a woman's stress and her IVF outcome. This is a surprising finding, as most recent studies support the link between stress and pregnancy.

We asked mind/body/fertility researcher Dr. Alice Domar to review the study and comment on its validity. Here is her response:

What Truly is the Relationship
Between Stress and IVF Outcome?

Alice D. Domar, Ph.D

There has been a huge amount of media interest in the recent publication in the *British Medical Journal* of the meta-analysis by Jacky Boivin, Ph.D., and her colleagues at Cardiff University in Wales. In this analysis, they pooled the results of 14 different studies that assessed the distress levels of women prior to an IVF cycle. They found that there was no significant relationship between distress and the pregnancy rate of that cycle. The authors concluded that women can stop worrying about their stress level since it won't have any impact on their ability to conceive.

My first response? I wish! I wish we knew it were definitive that stress had no impact on outcome, since that would take a lot of the guilt and worry that women have about how they are handling the psychological challenges of cycling.

The truth is, it's too soon to make any definitive statements about the relationship between stress and outcome. In fact, there have been 25+ studies on this topic, and most have shown a positive relationship. The biggest study—out of the Netherlands—did not, and this study constitutes about a fifth of the data in the meta-analysis. The Netherlands study has one major issue—few of the participants expressed any distress at all, which made it impossible to show any relationship.

The authors made note of this in their conclusion—culturally, women in that country tend to minimize their expression of distress, thus making it impossible to truly know what the relationship is. You also can't make any conclusions when you only assess distress at one point in time.

In the vast majority of the studies included, women were assessed once, and the time of the assessment varied from study to study. In fact, many women are highly optimistic prior to treatment and thus their true level of distress is masked. We presented a study at the reproductive medicine meeting last fall, where we actually measured distress not only prior to the cycle but also daily during the cycle. We actually found that the more distressed the women were prior to cycling, the *more* likely they were to conceive, but only if their distress level came down while cycling. In fact, women who were highly distressed prior to cycling but participated in a mind/body group and reported lower distress levels during their cycle had a 100 percent pregnancy rate.

So in conclusion, this meta-analysis provides us with more information about the stress/IVF relationship, but it is terribly premature to conclude that stress has no impact on outcome. We just don't know, and need more research to provide us with definitive answers.

Studies like this one are a double-edged sword. On the one hand, it's really great news to learn that stress may not impair a woman's odds of conception through IVF. The process is stressful enough without adding "stressing about stress" to the equation. On the other hand, it sends a problematic public health message. Saying that stress doesn't impact fertility because it doesn't impact IVF success is a bit like saying overeating has no impact on the obesity epidemic because it can be "cured" by techniques like gastric bypass surgery. There is a troubling tendency in our modern world to overlook the impact of our lifestyle practices because there's a miracle medical treatment that is "impervious" to them.

The Monkey Study

By now, you may be wondering what our position is on the question of whether stress causes infertility. Our answer is that in some women it does and in others it does not, but all women can benefit immensely from learning how to cope with stress and having a better understanding of where those stressors are coming from.

Let us explain. In our search for an answer to this question, we came upon an interesting piece of research that we often refer to as "The Monkey Study." So we're sharing it with you here.

Interestingly, monkeys tend to be pretty social animals. They get friendly with other monkeys, hang in groups, and show affection through grooming each other. It is believed that one particular species, the spider monkey, can die of loneliness when held in captivity and given little social interaction. In the particular study we are citing here (Bethea C. L. et al., 2005), monkeys that exhibited normal menstrual cycles were put under various forms of stress. First, they applied social stressors by separating the monkeys from their "friends." Second, they put the poor gals on a diet. And finally, the monkeys were stationed on a treadmill and forced to exercise.

Now doesn't that sound like the definition of a fertility patient? Isn't it true that during this process we end up being isolated from our friends, particular the Fertile Myrtle types who "oops" just got pregnant again? We can't eat or drink anything we want and between our jobs, personal commitments, and our TTC to do list, we feel like we are on a never-ending treadmill of stress?

As it turns out, the monkeys ended up dividing into three separate groups, with three distinct outcomes from this study. One group of monkeys showed no change in their menstrual activity through two separate cycles. This group was labeled as "highly stress resistant (HSR)" monkeys. The second group of monkeys ovulated normally during the first stress cycle, but did not ovulate in the second cycle. They were referred to as "medium stress resistant (MSR)." The final group of monkeys was labeled as "stress sensitive (SS)" because as soon as stressors were initiated, they shut down completely. They did not ovulate in either of the two stress cycles.

So what does this study say about the way we, as a society, handle stress? Is it possible that each of us has a different threshold of stress that can determine how our body will react in any given situation? I bet you have a friend or two who can take on 12 projects simultaneously, create gourmet dinners for 20, and go days without sleep and still look fresh as a daisy. Some of us are not fazed by stress, and some of us are a complete mess. One can argue about whether it's genetic, psychological, emotional, or something completely different, but perhaps the moral of the story is that some women, who are stressed, for whatever reason, just don't regularly ovulate. No ovulation, no pregnancy. Could it be another example of nature's "survival of the fittest?" When any particular individual's stress threshold is met, the body shuts down, preventing the proliferation of offspring.

Perhaps the silver lining in this whole study is the idea that stress can be regulated and a non-ovulating, stress-sensitive woman can do things to moderate her levels of stress. Think back to the ASRM position paper on stress. It encourages things like fertility-friendly exercise (see Fitness Guidelines in the next section), a good diet, and stress-reduction techniques like yoga, meditation, and acupuncture. We might not be able to eliminate stress, but there are things we can do to regulate it that will bring the body back into balance.

Let's go back to the monkeys and think about the stressors they were subjected to: diet, too much exercise, and isolation from their friends. Studies tell us that food deprivation can affect the menses. Think about women with eating disorders whose bodies shut down and they no longer ovulate. We also know that overexercising can affect the menses—Beth can tell you about that firsthand, from her own journey as an amenorrheac athlete compelled to run 40 miles a week. Yes, there are many different kinds of stresses that exist for the woman or couple dealing with infertility.

Another study interviewed couples about their experiences with the process of going through IVF (Imeson M et al, 1996). After sifting through the data, four key themes emerged:

1. They had intense feelings of social isolation, which were only intensified by the inappropriate responses of others.
2. They felt a sense of powerlessness and loss of control over many aspects of their lives.
3. Many described feeling stressed by the alternating cycles of hope and then disappointment that can come with each cycle.
4. They reported many life changes from physical to emotional and even mentioned changes in their relationships.

In the next chapter we will examine these themes in greater detail.

CHAPTER 6

Cleansing the Mind

In this chapter, we begin to look at the kinds of thoughts that challenge us when we're trying to conceive. As part of the Cleanse Lifestyle, we will ask you to a) identify negative thoughts, b) inquire into the nature of thoughts, and c) begin to explore the concept of Awareness, a powerful teaching from yoga that allows us to step into the flow of life in a radical way.

MENTAL TOXIN NO. 1: SOCIAL ISOLATION

Couples undergoing IVF mentioned social isolation as a recurring stressor in their treatment. We might wonder then if social isolation also contributes to the kind of stress that causes infertility? You know the kind of isolation we're talking about. The kind that says you can't attend your cousin's baby shower or meet your mommy friends at the park, or the kind that keeps you away from social activities at the office due to doctor appointments and concern over "sharing too much" about your personal "situation."

Could feelings of isolation impact our psychological well-being so much that it can actually impact our fertility? Some well-documented studies show psychosocial factors such as isolation and depression are the number one predictor of mortality in patients with heart disease and heart failure (Friedmann et al, 2006). Another study shows that people living in a culturally similar community who have the support of others actually have lower rates of heart disease.

Yes, the kind of social isolation that comes from being infertile can be a source of stress and even depression. There's no research yet on social isolation and infertility, but if depression can negatively affect IVF outcomes and social isolation causes depression, it makes sense that there could be a correlation. Remember, the lonely monkeys we mentioned earlier in the book. Therefore, it's important for gals trying to conceive to find and receive the appropriate support they need for this process. The question then becomes, what kind of support network or friends do *you* have?

If your friends are the Fertile Myrtle type or tell you to "just relax and it will happen"—just the kind of friends who participants in the study cited as causing stress for them—you may need to rethink your friendships. What you need are girlfriends who get it—and let us tell you, there are plenty of them out there.

Infertility affects one in eight women in the United States. Every time we sit down to a business meeting at Pulling Down the Moon, the person across the table inevitably shares a personal fertility story with us: "I went through it myself," or "my sister just had a baby after eight years of trying," or "my best friend just miscarried."

The problem is women just don't want to share, because they're not sure it's safe territory or an appropriate topic. As far as we've come in bringing social issues to the forefront of human consciousness, infertility is *still in the broom closet!* We hate to be the bearers of bad news, but if we don't give it to you straight, no one will.

Human reproduction is a primal instinct. Women, in particular, can feel hard-wired to bear a child or be a mother. Anthropologists tell us we are the gatherers and stokers of the home fires. As a result, many women will stop at nothing to accomplish the goal of having a baby, and when it doesn't happen, we sometimes feel ashamed, want to withdraw, or have the misperception that our bodies are broken.

Men, on the other hand, may come to this journey from a different perspective. While many men are completely supportive of their wives or partners, fertility can still be very closely linked to virility for them. We've all heard the braggadocio male—the one who announces that his wife is pregnant due to his strong swimmers or his "A-Team" or "his boys." Isn't it ironic that more than 30 percent of all infertility issues are due to the male factor? We share that statistic during some of our couples classes at Pulling Down the Moon and many of the guys look around the room like, "It ain't this male, so it must be you." If your spouse or partner is also in denial, remind them that it takes two.

On the other hand, we had a couple come to Pulling Down the Moon for our "Dealing with Disappointment" program, and the wife comforted the husband during the entire program as he cried his eyes out about the grief and disappointment he was feeling and his inability to talk about it with his male peers.

There are many things men can do to enhance their own fertility, including a visit to the urologist to check under the hood. A healthy diet that supports sperm production, a decrease in alcohol consumption, quitting smoking, wearing boxers instead of briefs, and refraining from "spanking the monkey" (masturbating) before and during their partner's ovulation period are also supportive techniques. One of the fertility doctors we work with at Fertility Centers of Illinois laughs when she tells the story about how this topic is approached with couples in her office. She says that most women can't imagine that their husband or spouse would be regular masturbators, so they often don't take her seriously when she mentions this during their initial consultation. The men, on the other hand, know exactly what she's talking about. Remember that a little bit of abstinence in this department can go a long way.

You can have the most wonderful spouse or partner on the planet, but that doesn't mean they make good "girlfriends." Remember if women are hard-wired to gather and men are hard-wired to hunt and fix things, most of us will be hard pressed to find a male partner who wants to hear our every thought, insecurity, idea, and emotion when it comes to trying to conceive. Girlfriends who are also trying to conceive, on the other hand, are a true gift!

Find support groups like those offered through Resolve, the AFA, or at your local fertility clinic. Be physically present. While online chatting or support groups can be nice, they can also lead to an enormous amount of unnecessary stress when you plug into the crazy lady whose story should be a made for TV movie or whose doctor was related to Mr. Hyde. When we wrote *Fully Fertile* a few years back, it was our intention that women everywhere could use the book as a way to create support groups in their local areas. The second edition of the book now contains a workbook and instructions on how to start a group near you. We are happy to report that Fully Fertile book clubs are popping up all over the place, so perhaps you'd like to start one, too.

It Takes a Village: Find Yours

Over the years, we've learned from our own personal experiences with infertility and our work at Pulling Down the Moon that the life of a gal trying to conceive can indeed be discouraging and lonely. It's easy for us to share our infertility stories with you now, two kids and many years later, but it wasn't that way in the beginning. Tami writes:

> *I didn't tell anybody I was trying to get pregnant. I didn't want to continually be asked about It, and I didn't want to feel like a failure at it. One of my close friends was having a devil of a time trying to get pregnant, and I remember being a mute when she brought it up. I somehow felt that if I didn't talk about it, it didn't really exist. To me, verbalizing the fact that I struggled with getting pregnant was like jinxing the whole process and, in my mind, I felt certain that if I spoke of it, I was sure to never get pregnant. It's funny how superstitious we get in times of crisis. Instead of reaching out, I retracted like a turtle in its shell. There is something profound that happens when you come out of your shell and become part of a group.*

In yoga, we often use the word sangha, which is a Sanskrit term referring to the idea that when liked-minded people come together, the power or intention of the group is magnified. We saw it for years in our Yoga for Fertility classes. Women who practiced the postures as a group and then came together for discussion every week felt supported and often healed by the group. Many got pregnant, many were able to move toward second solutions, and many told us that the yoga was a type of cleansing experience for them. One patient writes the following about her Yoga for Fertility experience:

> *"I have really enjoyed the current class and really look forward to it. It's like two hours of solace for me. I had miscarried two weeks before the class started and wasn't really looking forward to opening up and talking about my experience. Perhaps that's why I was so overly emotional on the first day and I just kept telling myself "I'm not ready to talk about this, I'm just not ready." But opening up that first day was what I really needed. It increases the load that one carries if you keep it all in. I wish I had started the class when I began my first two cycles, perhaps it would have made coping with the experience a lot easier – and I would have found a better outlet than eating my sorrows away on a Portillo's hot dog, fries and vanilla shakes!"*

The postures helped them cleanse their bodies on a physical level and the discussion and teachings of yoga helped cleanse them on a mental and emotional level. The women felt comforted in knowing that what they were feeling was not unique to them, that the trials and tribulations of trying to conceive were felt by many and that they weren't so "crazy" after all.

They learned from the group to look at their thoughts from an observer's point of view. In yoga, we challenged them to welcome their thoughts, feelings, and emotions rather than avoid them. We asked them to experience a bit of detachment and just acknowledge what they find. Rather than thinking, "I am broken and infertile," we asked them to observe their thoughts as though they were outsiders looking in. First, we asked them to look at those sitting next to them. Do they look broken and infertile? Next, we encouraged them to look at themselves. "Are you really broken and infertile?" we asked, "Or are you simply identifying with the feeling of being broken and infertile?" There is a huge distinction and, unfortunately, all too often we become identified with our thoughts. Sadly, we become what we think, and our perception becomes our reality. More on that later.

After we wrote *Fully Fertile*, we decided to conduct a pilot program at Pulling Down the Moon centered around the title. We envisioned hosting a weekly group that would read our book, follow the advice, and put it into practice in their lives. We hoped to track not only pregnancy outcomes but the overall changes each of the women went through as a result of integrating these holistic services into their lives. The Fully Fertile Book Clubs were not designed to be conducted like clinical trials; rather, they were an attempt to see if we could empirically say that the groups worked on some level in providing support, stress management tools, and a sense of community for its participants. You know: Could girlfriends really make a difference?

We put a notice in the tea room of our center and posted one online, asking for recruits who might be interested in participating in a new, 12-week Fully Fertile holistic book group. We recruited nine women of various ages and stages in their fertility treatment, each excited about trying something new and intrigued by the idea of adding a mind/body program to their treatment. Most of the women were going through medical treatment simultaneously; some had experienced multiple rounds of unsuccessful IVF; two chose not to do medical intervention at all; and one was experiencing secondary infertility.

When we wrote *Fully Fertile*, we felt it was important to include our own personal stories about our infertility journey in an attempt to connect with the reader. Similarly, in most of Pulling Down the Moon's mind/body classes, we ask participants to share as much as they feel comfortable sharing.

The stories are always moving—in some cases, they are even heroic. Every time a story is shared, there is a humble silence that moves over the class. There really is no way to describe the feelings in the room after that. Tears have been shed, the Kleenex box passed, anger expressed, and disappointments shared. We like to think of that time as the moment when grace enters the room and becomes a comfort to all of us.

MENTAL TOXIN NO. 2: LOSS OF POWER

By now, most of you reading this book have probably come to the conclusion that you are not a completely stress-resistant monkey. In addition, we're willing to bet that most of you probably do feel quite powerless during this process and that contributes greatly to your stress. Power, by definition, is the ability to control your environment or produce a desired effect, or have influence over others. The word power comes from the Old French word *pooir,* which means: to be able. When you are feeling powerless, you are feeling the opposite of able, which is "dis-able."

Where does this "able-ness" or "dis-ableness" come from? Some of you might claim that power comes from gaining knowledge through experiences, so the more experiences you have, the more power. Others might say that power comes from money, intelligence, or beauty. And still others might say that power is something you are born with. Let's be clear here. The kind of power we are talking about is not the kind that helps you command attention at a cocktail party or in interviews on national TV. We are talking about the kind of power that makes you feel as though you have some control over your own destiny. The kind of power that allows you to be happy in the face of adversity.

What if we told you that able-ness is your divine birthright, that everyone has the same ability to be powerful or control some aspects of their own destiny. Many people create feelings of being powerless by making the unconscious choice to be that way.

What is Unconscious Choice?

When we make a choice that we cannot remember making, it is an unconscious choice. Unconscious choices make us feel as though something, someone, or some power outside ourselves made those choices for us. As a result, we feel disconnected from the Source (our best selves) and believe we have an inability to change those choices. This attitude prevents us from being the creator or sculptor of our own lives and makes us feel as though we are apart from life's choices rather than a part of them.

The consequence of a powerless attitude is that we eventually start acting that way automatically. We do what powerless people do and have what powerless people have, which is a sense of lack in all areas of our lives. We essentially create what we are feeling. The antidote to feeling powerless is to make the *conscious* choice of acting powerfully. In this very moment, if you choose to be powerful, you will do the exact opposite of what powerless people do. Just because you feel powerless, it doesn't mean you are powerless. It only means you are identifying with that feeling at this point in time. You should question that feeling each and every time you feel it. Ask yourself, "What would a powerful person do in my situation?" What would a powerful person do when they are facing the challenges of infertility?

People who choose to be powerful make an attempt to do what powerful people do, act as powerful people act, and have what powerful people have—namely, health, happiness, prosperity, and abundance in all areas of their lives.

There is a sacred mantra in yoga that we would like you to chant every morning when you wake up, during the day when you think of it, and at night before you go to bed. Saying it to yourself or under your breath is completely acceptable.

The mantra is **AHAMBRAHMASMI**, which means:
I AM THE CREATIVE PRINCIPLE.

Remember, the mind is a very influential instrument, but too often we become its servant rather than its master. This is because the mind is such fertile breeding ground for all kinds of negative, powerless thoughts, and we believe that we are beholden to it. The mind needs to be trained like a wild stallion so it can serve us appropriately. Think of it as a mental detoxification. A mind that has been misused or untrained can become polluted by the negative, poverty-minded thinking of others who value unhappy and powerless thoughts more than they value happiness and thoughts of prosperity. When we begin to understand that happiness and prosperity are our birthright, only then can we see clearly the magnitude of power we hold within.

You Are What You Think—and I Think I'm Stressed and Powerless

We introduced a pretty bold concept in the previous section. We are saying that your unconscious mind has created a whole world for you and it, along with your conscious mind, aren't always the good guys. In yoga, much attention is paid to the mind/body/spirit connection and it is worth reiterating here. We're sure most of you have heard the saying, "You are what you eat." What if we told you, "You are what you think?"

We mentioned in the previous section that if you start to believe you are powerless, you will act powerless. Similarly, if you think or feel stress in your mental body, things will start to feel off kilter in your physical body, too. Your blood pressure might rise, your eating habits could change, your sleep become disrupted, and your mood might change. It's really quite remarkable. When a stressor presents itself, both the mind and the body are affected. We know this to be true from clinical studies showing that stress can lead to health conditions such as heart disease. Tami writes:

> I've been writing, talking, and teaching about the mind/body connection for years, but it really hit home for me when my 48-year-old husband Brian, who had previously been healthy as a horse, started complaining one night of pain in both of his arms. He was convinced it was from the heavy lifting he had done earlier in the day to reposition some furniture in the home office. When he turned gray and said he thought he might pass out, we got in the car and went straight to the emergency room. In no time at all blood panels had come back showing a high concentration of troponins which are the heart enzymes thrown off by the heart muscle when it is in distress. He was whisked away for an angiogram, which showed 100 percent blockage in one of his arteries, luckily a minor one. He received a stent and has since been in excellent physical health. The interesting thing is that Brian had no indicators for heart disease. He doesn't smoke, doesn't drink, is not overweight, eats fairly healthy, had borderline cholesterol numbers, and no one in his family has or had heart trouble. There is only one risk factor that Brian has, and that was his highly stressful job. It's a job that he enjoys, but it's still stressful, nonetheless. In fact, two years prior to the start of his new job, Brian and I both went to one of those Heart Check places where they take MRI- type photos of your arteries to make sure there was no indication of plaque buildup. We heard their commercials on the radio and thought it sounded like a great way to have early detection of any sort of issues. We applauded ourselves for being so proactive, especially when both of our tests came back clean. In my mind, this was a personal and classic example of how stress and anxiety can ultimately affect the physical body.

So if we are what we think, how do we train our mind to have thoughts that produce a more positive effect on the physical body? That's a tough one, but let's keep exploring.

What is a Thought?

By definition, a thought is what happens when we think or reason something. Scientists tell us that when an action takes place there is also a result. In this case, thinking is the action, and a thought is the result. This result could come in the form of a million different things. It could be the awareness of a feeling such as stress, fear, joy, love, or the result could produce a physical symptom such as insomnia, loss of appetite, or an addiction.

We know that we can't stop the process altogether. We will never stop the brain from thinking, so we can't just turn our brains off and say, "stop it." We really can't control our thoughts, either. A thought will be produced as the result of thinking. Ideally speaking, if we could somehow learn to control our thoughts, we just might be able to control our reactions and if that were the case, that would be a pretty powerful proposition.

Thoughts Have Energy

So if an action like thinking can produce a thought and, subsequently, the awareness of a feeling like stress, then there is power in the very act of thinking. In yoga, it is believed that this power is energy. Energy, as science describes it, is the ability to do work or the ability to make something happen. Remember that definition from physics class in high school? Scientists don't really know exactly what energy is, they just know how to describe its characteristics—that it's the ability to do work or make things happen.

In yoga it is believed that although you can't see it, every time you start thinking, you send energy out into the universe and that energy has a lot of power. Not only does the energy create a thought but it also is believed to attract other energies of a similar nature that sort of "hang around" you. We've all experienced being with someone who is always a complete downer, right? Being around them brings us down, too. Why? Because the power of their negative thought forms are sent out as energy attracting more negative thought forms and before you know it, you as the outsider, are standing there surrounded by so much negative energy and power that you can't help but feel like a party pooper yourself.

How about when you enter an old house and you are convinced it's haunted? Are there really ghosts? Nope, just the power of the energy left behind from the thought forms from everybody who ever lived in the house. In fact, Tami has made more than a few "house calls" clearing out so-called "ghosts" from people's homes. Move the energy, move the ghost. Get it?

So, what happens when you have thoughts like, "This is never going to happen," or "This body is completely broken," or "I am powerless?" Well, you send those toxic energies out into the world and attract a whole bunch more just like them. Since energy is the ability to make things happen, guess what you are in the process of doing? You are turning your mental thoughts into energy and helping create them in the physical world. As soon as you start to believe your thoughts (even if they are unconscious) and put emotional energy into them, you are manifesting them.

Try exercise No. 1 in Section 3
to help you understand how to manifest a different reality.

Thought form energy can also work to our advantage when we plant seeds of intention, send them out into the world and then watch them grow in front of your very eyes. Learning to channel your power in the right direction is critical in cleansing the mind. Watch what happens when you drop positive thoughts into your day by performing exercise No. 2 in the third section of this book.

MENTAL TOXIN NO. 3: RIDING THE ALTERNATING CYCLE OF HOPE AND DESPAIR

You've heard it said a thousand times, "Life is a series of ups and downs." What you may *not* readily see is that often we tend to be either in a state of complete happiness or in a state of complete despair and/or stress. The best place to be is right in the middle, a place of contentment. Unfortunately, the middle ground isn't very sexy. It doesn't bring about the euphoria of complete happiness nor the drama of feeling stressed and in despair. When someone asks you how you are, you may say, "I'm good" or "I'm a bit under the weather these days." We seldom say, "I am content." It's boring, nebulous, and sounds noncommittal.

Contentment, however, is quite the contrary. Contentment is not jump-for-joy happiness; nevertheless, it can be joyful. The joy might come from quiet moments, feeling connected, experiencing calm, feeling loved, or even being inspired by a great leader. Perhaps a better way of saying we should strive to be content is to say that we should learn to increase our overall positivity. Over-the-moon happiness is not the only path to a joy-filled life.

Staff psychologists from FCI, Dr. Marie Davidson and Caitlin Roche explain that they often tell fertility patients to focus on what they call "The Neutral Zone." Dr. Davidson goes on to describe this space: "Imagine it's a room that's very nicely furnished, has a nice color on the walls, and feels very safe. You have complete control in this room. The thoughts you have in this space don't promise too much about the future or focus on any part of the past. The thoughts inside this room aren't scary, either."

Part of the mental detox program is learning not to live in the extremes of life. Don't think for a moment that your good day and good luck will last forever, and don't be fooled into thinking your bad luck or difficult situations will, either. What is it the Bible says, "This too shall pass?" Don't be too quick to float on cloud nine because you had 25 eggs retrieved for your IVF. Similarly, don't be disappointed because those 25 eggs turned into only one viable embryo for transfer. Ups and downs, highs and lows, they are all a part of life so learn to embrace them. We only know what extreme happiness feels like because we have experienced its opposite which is extreme sadness.

So you see life is really all about learning how to cope with extremes. When we are feeling down, it's the memory or hope of happiness that can often pull us through. The trick is learning how to stand right in that middle ground, watching the highs and lows and being able to come away with a sense of contentment and positivity.

Try exercise No. 3 in Section 3,
entitled, "It's My Story," graciously provided by Dr. Marie Davidson.

The Law of Opposites

Isn't it true that you understand what cold feels like because you also have experienced hot? You know what darkness is because you've seen the light of day and, thus, know the difference? In yoga philosophy and Oriental Medicine alike, it is believed that the universe is expressed through a series of opposites. The universe hums along, giving ground to two extremes or opposites that are able to coexist in perfect harmony and even transmute into one another.

When your yoga teacher tells you to "find your center," she is really saying, "Go inside and find the balance between the two extremes that already exist within you." In order for you to understand that you are stressed, you must have experienced a time of peace. Can you go inside and remember what peace feels like? Peace is simply a state of being. Nobody delivers it to you on a platter, and no matter how many times you may be told to "relax," the feeling of peace cannot be captured and placed in a jar and handed to you.

Sure, you can come to a place like Pulling Down the Moon and experience soft music, aromatherapy, and a caring practitioner to help you feel better; ultimately, though, you are the peace bringer and nobody else.

Have you ever known someone who was madly in love with their spouse and then they get divorced and they can't stand each other? Tami's grandmother used to always say the closest thing to love is hate, and it couldn't be more accurate. That's because in order to know you love someone you have to know what hate feels like, and both of those feelings have existed inside you. When you feel scorned by your lover, the small bit of hate that exists within the love grows larger. The more you send energy into the small spec of hate, the larger it grows, until you find yourself feeling the opposite of love. Interestingly, even when you hate someone, there is a speck of love that still exists. In order to understand this concept more fully and give you some visual direction, consider the Tai Chi symbol found in Oriental Medicine. While this symbol was first introduced in our previous book, *Fully Fertile*, it deserves a bit of further study now. Let's call it the Tai Chi 201 lesson.

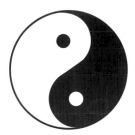

This symbol is meant to represent the duality that exists in nature, the dark and the light, the Yin and the Yang, or the male and the female. Notice that the line between the dark and light is not straight and predictable. It's just like a metaphor for life: it swirls a bit between the black and white. Also notice that within the light exists a black dot and within the black exists the white. This is meant to express the idea that all opposites contain pieces of each other. As we said before, they are able to transmute properties of themselves into the opposite.

This is a very important concept to understand and one that is imperative for helping cleanse the mind. If our thoughts are negative, or if we are feeling particularly stressed or overwhelmed, that means we have also known all the opposite of these things. Similarly, wherever there is destruction, the seed of creation has also been planted.

Perhaps you have heard a story of how a simple man became a millionaire in times of economic difficulty or depression despite the horrific environment or conditions surrounding him. This is an example of how the seed of opportunity exists within the most adverse conditions. In order for something new to be created, you should make room for something else to be destroyed. This is not to say that in order for a birth to occur you must experience a death. It is a symbolic birth and a symbolic death. You might be able to point to ways your struggle in trying to conceive has led to incredible opportunities or insights that you might not have otherwise had. We, the authors, have often said that without having experienced infertility and loss ourselves, Pulling Down the Moon would never exist. Perhaps we are the classic example of what Greek mythology and Carl Jung would call "The Wounded Healer." Through hardship and loss, an opportunity for us to fulfill a dream and help other people was realized.

So remember, an important step in your journey toward cleansing the mind is beginning to understand that no matter how difficult this journey has become, the seed of opportunity (or the opposite of despair, frustration, you name it) also exists. This is not meant to sound like *rah, rah* cheerleader, "You go girl you can do it," type of advice. Nor is it meant to suggest that just by thinking positive thoughts you will get pregnant. It does, however, challenge you to play an active role in how you think and what you think regarding your fertility journey. That is the cleansing process. It also encourages you to see that speck of light or opportunity within every challenge.

Some days may be pitch perfect for us, and we feel as though life is in three-part harmony, but most days, we struggle to find the balance between happy and sad, good and evil, stress and peace, hot and cold, being asleep and being awake.

Increasing Positivity

We recently attended a lecture by Dr. Barbara Frederickson, a researcher from the University of North Carolina who spoke about studies currently being done on the benefits of positivity. It seems that learning how to self-generate positive emotions can transform us. In fact, The National Institute of Health (NIH) is currently looking at how positive emotions can promote health and longevity by changing the gene expression at the DNA level. In the lecture we attended by Dr. Frederickson, she made a series of key points:

1. POSITIVITY OPENS US. Positive emotions act on human beings like the sun on flowers. Researchers found through MRI that the opposing influences of positive and negative states of mind extend to perceptual encoding in the visual cortices. Positive emotions changed how open subjects were to visual information. Dr. Frederickson argues that this opening effect extends widely to include more possibilities, more creativity, more resilience, better performance, better problem solving, more oneness/trusting, and better negotiating. These are big claims, but there's a good deal of research to justify them. Beth writes:

Remaining Open

"I never knew that things exploded…
I only found it out when I was down upon my knees…
looking for my life." ~ *GEORGE HARRISON*

Loss is a dirty word in our culture. Loss is a form of the word "lose," and from very early on we are culturally conditioned to shun loss and to view it as a form of personal failure. Yet, time and again at Pulling Down the Moon, I have spoken to women who found that the loss and disappointment they experienced through the process of infertility actually brought them a sense of spaciousness and authenticity. When we lose something we didn't plan on losing, all of our assumptions about life and justice are called into question. We are forced, as I like to tell my yoga students, to step out of the groove of Plan A (the way we thought things would be) into Plan B (the way things are).

Recently I was riding home from work with our wise-beyond-her-years Chicago admin/receptionist Jenny when our conversation turned to coping with loss. This had not been an easy winter for Jenny, who had lost most of her earthly belongings in an apartment fire that left her homeless in February. During the catastrophic event and the aftermath, Jenny remained steady and positive, giving support and compassion to our patients while maintaining an impressively professional demeanor in her work. Everyone at Pulling Down the Moon was inspired.

Since I had been noodling about writing about loss in my head, I thought it would be useful to ask Jenny about the fire and the strategies she used for recovery. I thought it would provide a foil for the losses I could write about from personal experience (miscarriages and a stillbirth) and for the kinds of losses we encounter at our Center. These are largely emotional losses—hopes and dreams of pregnancy, failed cycles, miscarriages and stillbirth. At times these losses are coupled with the loss of resources, in cases where couples have paid out of pocket for unsuccessful treatments, but they are largely emotional. Jenny's loss was concrete—literally, valuable possessions as well as priceless mementos that were completely destroyed by a bolt from the blue.

"I kept telling myself that there is a bigger picture," she said. "It was the old saying that 'Things happen for a reason' that gave me strength. I really focused on staying positive and looking for the good that might come."

If you smell a cliche here, keep reading. Jenny's next words were profound.

"I think it's human nature to contract when we experience loss. We contract around the pain. We avoid situations that remind us of our loss and we try to avoid the emotions—sadness, anger and envy—that come when our life seems to be in shambles compared to those around us. More than anything I tried to remain open—to emotions, to help from others and even to situations that could be painful."

As Jenny shared her experiences of loss and healing, I was instantly struck by their similarity to my own journey. When my first full-term pregnancy ended in a stillbirth of a little girl at 38 weeks, I received one strong message from the universe: STAY OPEN. Take every condolence call, accept every offer of comfort from friends, eat every casserole that is delivered and, above all, cry every tear that I need to cry. For a very introverted and private person (at least before the creation of Pulling Down the Moon) this was indeed a radical strategy. My entire being wanted to crawl in a hole and avoid contact with others and with my pain.

In Jenny's case, this call to open was an intuition. In my own case, I believe the message came through my yoga practice. The simple practice of stretching that has been part of my life for so many years kept calling to me to use the same techniques that keep my body healthy to heal my mind. If you've ever been a beginning yogi, you know it can be an uncomfortable business at first to stretch tight muscles. Yet, with practice, the discomfort eventually releases and gives way to spaciousness and calm. This holds true for emotional challenges, too. When we choose to stay open and experience our loss we can actually release pain and suffering. When we "close" around these painful emotions, we may not ever let them go. In fact, we will often consciously or unconsciously go to great lengths to avoid the aspects of life that trigger past trauma and in doing so greatly circumscribe the scope of our experience.

There seems to be an energetic rule in play here, and the similarity of Jenny's and my experience drove this home. In the face of loss, rather than constriction, we must look for ways to open. Begin with a simple physical practice of stretching and breathing. Find support where you can tell your story and cry tears with people who understand. Eat the casserole. Like George Costanza from 'Seinfeld', do the opposite of what feels comfortable and stretch instead of hunker.

These are not easy words of advice. Yet, there is a promise of courage and self-discovery in them. Staying open and finding the light in the darkness can transform us in profound ways.

2. POSITIVITY TRANSFORMS US. There is a very long cranial nerve known as the vagus nerve, which runs from deep in the brain, through the neck and all the way down to the abdomen. The vagus nerve has a number of branching nerves which come into contact with many other body parts including the heart, lungs, voicebox, stomach, and ears. The vagus nerve carries incoming information from the nervous system to the brain, providing details about what the body is doing, and it also transmits outgoing information which governs a range of reflex responses. The vagus nerve is believed to be the antidote to the "fight-or-flight" response in the body because it slows down the heart rate and can regulate the heart on a breath-by-breath level. Since it wanders down toward the diaphragm, deep, rhythmic, belly breathing can stimulate this nerve and send positive "relaxation" signals to the brain. Changes in vagal tone are likely to have major effects on multiple body systems including stress, mood, heart, digestion, inflammation, and immune function. As an aside, the vagus controls voice muscles—maybe one of the reasons why the sound of a person's voice can tell us so much about them and their existing levels of mental stress or discomfort.

High vagal tone is good because it means the body is working to slow down the heart when exhaling and speeds up the heart when inhaling, which leads to better health. Low vagal tone has been associated with social anxiety and generalized anxiety/worry problems. Dr. Frederickson's research shows that meditation and relaxation methods seem to increase vagal tone and activity (Fredrickson, Cohn et al., 2008).

Craniosacral Therapy

There is one aspect related to this, which is quite basic, too: The vagus nerve, cranial nerve number 10, the longest of the 12 cranial nerves, exits the skull through the jugular foramen, along with two other cranial nerves. It's located between the occiput and the temporal bone behind the ears. The vagus travels down into the belly and controls all the important functions in the body, such as respiration, digestion, etc. When people are stressed, and breathing shallowly, the jugular foramen gets pinched off, causing distress. Restoring proper cranial nerve function and allowing parasympathetic function to take over and help restore whole body coherence and good functioning is one of the main goals of the biodynamic craniosacral therapy offered by many holistic practitioners today.

It might be easy to talk about increasing positivity and its potential value with regard to infertility, but how do you actually make it happen? What's the practical application?

Interestingly, Dr. Frederickson's research showed that practicing Loving Kindness Meditation over time produced positive emotions, which, in turn, created substantial increases in a wide range of personal resources. For example, people felt more mindful, a greater purpose in life, more supported by their social networks, and a decrease in the symptoms of illness. In turn, these increments in personal resources increased their feeling of life satisfaction (contentment) and reduced symptoms of depression.

Dr. Frederickson isn't the only one who believes a meditation practice can increase a person's overall happiness. Jon Kabat-Zinn, co-developer of Mindfulness-Based Stress Reduction, collaborated with Davidson and others (Davidson et al., 2003) to examine the brain and immunological effects of beginning a meditation practice.

Volunteers in the study were required to attend a mindfulness-based stress-reduction (MBSR) workshop, which also required a daily practice of guided meditation lasting about one hour. It was shown that anxiety levels were significantly reduced in the meditation group and that left-side anterior brain function was increased, which has been repeatedly linked to greater positive emotions. Meditators also showed a more robust and effective immune response to a flu vaccine administered at the end of the training period, and the strength of this response was related to the magnitude of the left-sided anterior brain activation.

Most empirical work on meditation has been focused on mindfulness meditation, also called insight meditation, which has buddhist roots. Loving Kindness Meditation is a related technique used to increase feelings of warmth and caring for yourself and others. Similar to other meditation practices, it includes sitting in quiet contemplation with the eyes closed while focusing on the sound or movement of the breath.

Whereas mindfulness encourages participants to focus on the present moment in an open and nonjudgmental way, LKM involves directing your attention to the region of the heart and then evoking warm and tender feelings about another person or persons close to you. You are then asked to extend those warm feelings first toward yourself (self-compassion) and then outward to an ever expanding circle of others. The idea is to broaden your feelings of tenderness and build upon it.

The primary goal with any meditation practice is to learn about the nature of the mind and dispel false assumptions about the sources of happiness (Dalai Lama & Cutler, 1998). It is believed that insights gained through a meditation practice shift conscious and unconscious beliefs and can shift a person's basic outlook on themselves in relation to others. While the positivity research specifically uses LKM techniques, it is our belief that any mindful, daily meditation practice will produce similar results.

We'll explore some meditation techniques later in the book that we hope you will adopt as part of your cleanse program.

MENTAL TOXIN NO. 4: LIFE CHANGES RESULTING FROM INFERTILITY ARE DRIVING ME CRAZY

Cycles, Patterns, and Change

"Change is inevitable. Growth is optional." ~ John C. Maxwell

The universe is dynamic and always changing. Sometimes the change is infinitesimal and beyond our detection, but often we can see this change with our own eyes. We know what the changing seasons look like, we understand planetary motion, lunar phases, the high and low tide, weather systems, shifting winds, the flow of the river, erosion, our moods, our bodies and even the birth, aging and death of living things. To say we want to have some control over the changes in life is like asking the earth to shower us with rain only every other Saturday. All of nature seems to subscribe to the same idea: life flows, time passes, and things change no matter how hard we may wish they stay the same.

Yogis like to say that we are not breathing the earth; the earth is breathing us, through a constantly changing series of inhales and exhales. It's a philosophical concept, for sure, but change is also scientific. Mathematicians might refer to this condition by illustrating it with a graph that shows a sine curve. You've seen these graphs before—they peak above and below the base line like a series of waves. This pattern occurs often in nature as sound waves, light waves, and even ocean waves that keep changing and moving. Change in life, and in this universe, is completely natural; it's our resistance to this change and our clinging to the familiar that is unnatural. Since change is the only constant in life, we have to get used to the idea that letting go of our fear of the unknown allows us the opportunity to create space and the potential to birth something new and potentially greater in our lives. We couldn't say this more poetically than the television show *Grey's Anatomy* did in a September 23, 2010 episode:

Opening Voiceover

Every cell in the human body regenerates on average every seven years. Like snakes, in our own way we shed our skin. Biologically, we are brand new people. We may look the same—we probably do; the change isn't visible at least in most of us—but we are all changed completely forever.

Closing Voiceover

When we say things like people don't change, it drives scientists crazy because change is literally the only constant in all of science. Energy, matter, it's always changing, morphing, merging, growing, dying. It's the way people try not to change that's unnatural. The way we cling to what things were instead of letting them be what they are. The way we cling to old memories instead of forming new ones. The way we insist on believing despite every scientific indication, that anything in this life is permanent. Change is constant. How we experience change, that's up to us. It can feel like death, or it can feel like a second chance at life. If we open our fingers, loosen our grips, go with it, it can feel like pure adrenaline. Like at any moment we can have another chance at life. Like at any moment we can be born all over again.

Everyday, universal patterns can be used as important tools in understanding the cycles of life. By studying the seasons, for instance, we can understand the nature of life itself. We are born in the spring, we bloom in the summer, we become dormant in the fall, and we die in the winter. Some religions and cultures would say we are "reborn" in the spring just like the trees, and the cycle continues. The world is constantly changing.

Let's now return to the idea of ridding ourselves of mental toxicity by looking at this intelligence the universe has given us and drawing some of our own conclusions.

First, if there are indeed laws of nature that show how the world is constantly changing and flowing, there is little we can do to change it. The world will keep on humming and flowing and moving the way it is meant to regardless of what we think or do. Our microcosmic selves are a part of that macrocosmic flow. It's exactly as the quote at the beginning of this chapter states, "Change is inevitable," and we are just a part of the total flow of the universe. In yoga, we use the Sanskrit word *rita* to describe this sacred order or universal flow.

Along with humming and flowing and doing what it needs to do, the universe did play one small trick on us humans. It gave us free will. But in the process, we often fall into the trap of assuming we can control most of what happens to us simply by changing our actions or the choices we make. While we can certainly influence the outcome of our personal future by the choices we make, we cannot change it completely. For example, you have the free will to jump out of an airplane without a parachute, but the laws of the universe dictate that death will likely be the result. Now if you get yourself a parachute and some sky diving lessons, you have contributed whatever amount you can to the equation and the ratios have changed. The result might be a thrilling and safe jump.

Most often, there is very little we can do to change what will happen to us in life. We do our best to make good decisions through the free will we have been given but, ultimately, we are pawns in the universe's game of chess. So while it is difficult controlling what changes in our life, the one thing we can control is our reaction to this change. Our reaction to life's events is what brings about *karma*. For those who really don't understand what karma is, the word can be pretty onerous. Until we have a chance to look at it more in depth, let's just call karma our "predispositions" in life for now.

The Value of Awareness

Albert Einstein once said the definition of insanity was doing the same things over and over again and somehow expecting the result will be different. Sometimes, we just can't see the insanity of our ways. This is where it becomes important to have awareness. Awareness becomes an incredibly powerful mind-cleansing tool because we are able to see the insanity of patterns, habits, reactions, and predispositions. We acknowledge that often there is little we can do to change our difficult situation or the luck that has been handed to us. We are honest with ourselves and see if our own actions resulted in a reaction that is unwanted. Similarly, we can look at difficult situations and our reaction to them to see how our own habits and patterns begin to form. This kind of self-study (*Svadyaya*) gives us a clue as to how we might react and respond in all difficult situations that come our way in life, not just the current one.

When we are challenged by a situation, consciousness, or the thinking brain, goes through the mental exercise of reasoning and trying to understand why something difficult has happened. In the process, we might be feeling sad, mad, victimized, or angry. We have a thought and a corresponding reaction, which could be expressed as an emotion. As these emotions start to bubble up to the surface, Awareness is present, but it is clouded by our thinking brain and by our emotions.

From the yoga perspective, if we are able to step into Awareness, we will be able to welcome our emotions rather than fight against them. This acceptance of "what is" and the universal flow of energy can create a feeling of surrender within us that makes us feel as though we are a part of life. It begins the detox process from the inside out by ridding the mind of some of the negative emotions and feelings that do not serve us and allows us to see life in a different way. It's like standing on top of a mountain and having a view of the whole village rather than standing on the street and trying to stand on our tip-toes to see what restaurant is a block away.

Now try exercise No. 4 in Section 3
in the chapter on Finding Awareness.

The Deeper Practices

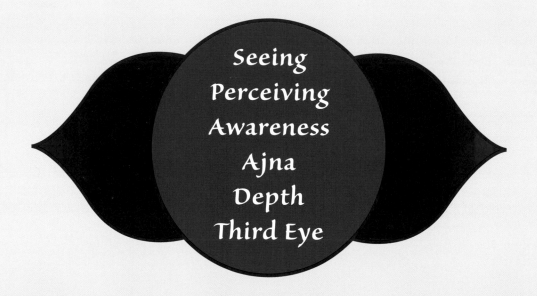

Seeing
Perceiving
Awareness
Ajna
Depth
Third Eye

Are You Ready?

CHAPTER 7

The Karma Component

In the previous chapter, we mentioned karma and promised to revisit it in a bit more depth. The truth is, karma could easily be its own book, and the interpretation of it can vary slightly from culture to culture, religion to religion or philosopher to philosopher. We thought it most important to explore karma in a way that would be accessible to our readers as a mind-cleansing tool in the tradition of yoga.

Karma really isn't a very complex term, but it can become complex because it is often misunderstood. It is not the law of getting even or "an eye for an eye." Rest assured, there is no karma police out there in the world watching your every move and waiting to handcuff you with some scary punishment. Karma doesn't discriminate. It doesn't like Fertile Myrtle or your pregnant girlfriend more than you.

Karma is the law of causation, the idea that you reap what you have sown, you get back what you put in. If you put love and forgiveness out into the world, love and forgiveness will find its way back to you. If you are constantly chanting the mantras of stress and worry, stress and worry will find you. Cause and effect, action and reaction is really what karma is all about.

The idea of karma has been around for ages but sometimes we don't even call it that. Sigmund Freud, the father of modern-day psychology, used free association in the hopes of creating a catharsis or emotional cleanse that would help move an experience or memory from the unconscious mind to the conscious mind. It was his belief that once these experiences can be processed and are no longer repressed the healing can begin.

While Freud did not call it such, the technique of becoming aware of the thoughts and beliefs in our unconscious minds is a way to help neutralize karma. Karma is generally created because of the intense emotion we feel surrounding an event. Emotions such as anger, jealousy, resentment, and hatred lead to negative actions, speech, or thoughts. The funny thing is, you can't hide from karma by deciding to ignore the thoughts, feelings, or experiences within you either. Even inaction can trigger a cause-and-effect reaction. For example, not doing your duty or not coming to the defense of helpless people also has karmic results.

It might be helpful to think of karma as that for which you have a predisposition rather than as some sort of law of retribution or punishment. For example, if you know you are prone to jealous or spiteful thoughts, it is useful to understand that karma might fire as a result of these thoughts. Sometimes it's not easy seeing our own predispositions, but self-study, honesty, and heightened awareness can help. Importantly, there is not a simple one-to-one correspondence between your actions and the result. It is impossible to know how the flow of karma will affect your life but it *is* possible to know that the universe works in perfect harmony, and that while you have free will to perform actions that create karma, you also have the opportunity to help neutralize difficult karma. We say you can neutralize karma rather than "get rid of it" because karma is like a debt each of us owes. Sooner or later the debt must be paid.

Get Back to Me When It All Makes Sense

When you feel ready to have a baby and the universe just isn't cooperating, it's easy to start asking those existential questions like, "Why me?" or "What did I do to deserve this?" Over the years at Pulling Down the Moon, more than a few women have asked us if infertility is some sort of punishment for past behavior or an attempt by God, the universe, or some cosmic force to teach a lesson or get even. We hope this discussion on cleansing your karma will shed some light on the situation, at least from a yogi's perspective.

First, and most importantly, you must understand what karma is and what it is not. We're not trying to beat a dead horse here, but let's review one more time. Karma is the law of causation. It is *not* an eye for an eye and a tooth for a tooth.

For example, if you steal $100 from someone, karma does not mean that $100 will be stolen from you. Going back to the law of causation, similar to the law of physics, karma basically says that for every action there is a reaction. The intensity or emotional response to the action is what creates karma.

Going back to our previous example: If the $100 you stole creates hardship, pain, and suffering for the victim and guilt for you, then all of that mental energy everybody is creating puts the karmic wheel in motion. The same karmic wheel is set in motion when you do something good and feel love and joy as a result. In this case, the emotional energy is very positive but it still creates karma. So to the yogi, karma is neither good nor bad, it is merely a constantly burning fire fueled by our actions and emotional energy. The quickest way to neutralize karma is by dousing the fire. If someone hurts you, send them love and blessings. Splash! You've just doused the flame. If, instead, you call that same person names and spread nasty rumors about them, you've set off a whole new chain of karmic events.

Let's explore a few misconceptions we have seen at Pulling Down the Moon during one-on-one sessions with patients going through infertility.

Let's say for instance, someone tells us they had an abortion when they were 20. The choice was very difficult. It felt at the time like a decision that would determine the success or failure of their life. After much debate and soul searching, the patient decided to terminate the pregnancy. Fast forward 15 years later, this same woman is struggling with her fertility. She can't help but feel and actually tells us that this is some sort of "karmic retribution" for her past actions. Is it? Yogis might argue that the biggest hurdle in this example is the woman's own emotional response to the event, her attitude, and her willingness to forgive herself. Morality or immorality aside, a large part of karma is having compassion for oneself and realizing that sometimes we did the best we could based on the information we had at the time.

Not all karma that could occur in this lifetime has to manifest. The stronger, more intense patterns will manifest as opposed to the weaker. For instance, karma is affected by attitude. If you say I'm bad, I deserve it, or I'll never have a child, you may actually be drawing out the more difficult pieces of karma. It is best to draw on the positive attitudes rather than the negative. Remember, karma is not fatalistic. If you are experiencing infertility in this lifetime, it means your cup of karma includes challenges with conception; it doesn't mean it's never going to happen or that it is your destiny.

As a result, you should feel free to get rid of any guilt you've been carrying around with regard to your fertility and past experiences or bad behavior. If your bad behavior is creating a great deal of emotion or feelings of sadness within you, however, it would be wise to try and neutralize some of these feelings by cleansing your karma.

Ways to Neutralize/Cleanse Difficult Karma

It is possible to help neutralize a piece of challenging karma. The first step is having awareness. Here are some other helpful suggestions:

1. Find Awareness, take a deep breath, and do the right thing at the right time. Admit when you are wrong and ask for forgiveness.
2. Send love and blessings to both your friends and your enemies, even if it is simply through your prayers and meditations.
3. Do something nice for your enemy.
4. Pray or meditate, asking the powers that be to neutralize the emotion you are feeling regarding a challenging piece of karma.
5. Do something good for somebody and expect nothing in return. If you do something with the expectation of reward (even good karma points), you will only create more karma for yourself when your expectations of reward are not met.
6. Seek the counsel of a priest, rabbi, minister, swami, psychologist, or spiritual guide who can help you rid some of the emotions surrounding karmic events.
7. Stop being so emotional. Trust the flow of the universe and its ever changing nature. Surrender to the idea that everything is exactly as it should be.
8. Change your attitude to draw in more positive energy.
9. Look in the mirror, note your own imperfections; love and forgive yourself anyway.

As a disclaimer we should note that just because you create good karma with the intention of having a baby, don't expect the universe to look at it that way. It may put your good karma toward keeping you healthy or getting you that promotion you've always wanted, or making you feel more content. In other words, you can't dictate where you want the karma to go, but trust that the universe has your back, and surrender to it. That might be the single most important thing you can do to earn good karma!

WAKING UP TO AWARENESS

We established in the previous section of the book that it is very easy to become what you think you are. The next step and deeper practice of cleansing the mind is to understand the difference between our conscious minds and our Awareness. You will note that in this section we will be using a capital "A" in the word Awareness as we would for a deity such as God, Buddha, Jesus, Zeus, Moses, or hundreds of others. It is meant to remind us that when we tap into Awareness we are tapping into our highest selves, something sacred and holy.

Let's begin by first gaining a better understanding of the conscious mind.

Our conscious mind is what we might call our thinking brain. We experience the world through our senses and then make judgments based on our beliefs or convictions. We then feel emotions accordingly. Think about what we are saying in terms of the senses. You only think someone is beautiful because you see them with your eyes and then make a judgment about their level of beauty. Your opinion is merely your opinion because someone else may think that your Prince Charming is a real dog. You, however, base your judgment on your perception of beauty and your comparison of its opposite: ugliness. We first use the senses to gather information for the conscious mind and then, because we make a judgment based on intellect, opinion, or experience, we process this information like a computer.

Remember the movie *Shallow Hal,* where Jack Black can only see inner beauty and ends up falling in love with a seemingly unattractive woman? What if we had no eyes and had to base beauty on a feeling instead of on a judgment made by our eyes? By closing our eyes, we have to open up other senses. Maybe we would open up our ears to hear clearer or our noses to smell better.

But what if we were like little turtles that lived inside our shells and had no physical senses at all? We would have to rely on something else in order to know if someone was beautiful. We would have to intuit how that person makes us feel or the "vibes" they send out into the world. If they make us feel good, we might consider them beautiful. If they make us feel bad, we would likely consider them less attractive. You've heard it said that everyone is beautiful in their own way, but our conscious minds make decisions based on information given and then processed by our senses. Our senses ultimately shroud our ability to see clearly. As a result, we make judgment calls every day of our lives based on thoughts from our mind and the information gathered by our senses.

Think of your senses gathering information and then uploading it to your conscious mind, which then acts like a computer. The mind computes a thought or judgment, then spits it out for us to believe. Most of us cannot recognize that we hold a secret treasure inside of us called Awareness. If we were to rid ourselves of our senses, and the judgments made by the mind, we would be left with just Awareness. Awareness just sits peacefully and watches everything happening as though it was viewing a movie on a picture screen. It sees our dramas and is interested. It can laugh at our comedies and cry with our tragedies but, in the end, Awareness knows that it is observing the theater of our minds. It exists in the perfect state of being as a detached but empathetic observer.

The Bible might say Awareness is Yahweh—"I Am Who Am." It's the exact middle of the Tai Chi symbol or the middle channel (Sushumna) in yoga because it represents perfection, balance, and the middle ground. We talked previously about avoiding the extreme highs and lows of life by striving to be in the middle, which is a place of contentment. That is where Awareness lives. It doesn't act, it doesn't react, it doesn't like or dislike; it just observes and witnesses and experiences with complete detachment and content. When something good happens, Awareness watches us feel happy. When something bad happens, Awareness watches us feel sad. It is able to transcend the nature of opposites.

Let's say that lately you are only able to experience one pair of opposing emotions—sadness. You just can't experience joy right now. In cases where you feel stuck in an extreme feeling or emotion, you need some tools for becoming "unstuck." Here are three for your infertility cleansing tool belt:

THREE STEPS FOR BECOMING UNSTUCK

1. CONNECT WITH THE OPPOSITE: Let's say that you are feeling really sad. The first thing you must acknowledge is that joy is still within you. Remember that joy is the opposite of sadness, and every opposite has a speck of the other extreme within it. Next, you must try to connect with that little speck of joy within the sadness and try to make it bigger. You can do this in a number of ways, such as listening to music that makes you happy or being around joy-filled people. It will be therapeutic for you to be in the energy of their thoughts and see what you can learn or observe and to notice how it makes you feel to be exposed to joy.

2. CONNECT WITH A SPIRITUAL GURU: Having a living guru or spiritual teacher can also be a cleansing process. These souls have the ability to absorb the energy of your sadness without snuffing out their own joy. They transmit more positive energy to you than you are able to transmit negative energy to them. If you don't have a spiritual teacher, don't fret. As the saying goes: When the student is ready, the teacher will appear. In the meantime, read inspirational biographies, go to lectures given by innately joyful individuals, visit your church or temple, meditate or pray.

3. SERVE OTHERS: Another technique for finding joy is through service. Find another individual who needs help in some way and serve them. If you cannot create joy within yourself, you might be able to create joy in someone else, and since the energy of joy is contagious you might be surprised at how your own feelings begin to shift.

MAKING DECISIONS BASED ON PAST EXPERIENCES

Many women who come for treatment at Pulling Down the Moon share with us very toxic memories they hold within. Some have experiences of miscarriage or stillbirths. Others have had painful memories of an unsuccessful IVF cycle. Still others come with heavy hearts from a death they experienced in their family or from abuse they knew as a child. Psychology tells us that often memories from our past can influence our future. In yoga, we call some of these experiences *samskaras,* or "scars" from the past. Our samskaras might make us do certain things, avoid others, or repeat bad behaviors.

Human beings are all the same: We want to avoid situations, people, or places that cause us pain. Once thrown from the horse, it can be very difficult and often painful getting back in the saddle. We see this so often in women who have not been successful with an IVF cycle or in those who have experienced a loss. Often there is no opportunity or forum to help a woman grieve the loss of a child, pregnancy, or failed cycle.

In these cases, it is very difficult to put closure on these devastating events and move forward or even think about trying again. Even though the reward could be the birth of a baby they so desperately want, for such women the idea of starting over again with a new cycle can, at times, be painful and feel overwhelming. It can take more than a leap of faith; it can take a tremendous amount of courage and trust that they won't get hurt again if they try.

While there are never any guarantees, you have to take your own risk/reward assessment and determine whether the toxic thoughts created by your mind are limiting your ability to actually achieve the reward you seek. If it is determined that the risk is too great, you must also be content in knowing that the reward will never be achieved, either. Can you live happily and joyfully without this reward? If not, you must take the risk.

Bringing Awareness into our past can often help us understand our samskaras and can be an important part of the cleansing process, as Awareness helps detox our future as well as provide us with greater wisdom and clarity. Beth writes:

Rambo Fertility Yoga

For those of you who do not know my story, I was one of those gals who unfortunately needed seven years and five pregnancies to get two children. One of my losses was particularly difficult—a stillbirth in the 38th week of a pregnancy. For this book, Tami asked me to write about how I managed to make it through the subsequent pregnancy, which resulted in the arrival of my first son, Jackson, one month before Pulling Down the Moon opened its first center in Chicago. She probably thought that I might have some words of wisdom for dealing with the anxiety and, yes, I would call it post-traumatic stress that are part of a subsequent pregnancy after such a loss.

I don't. You see, I didn't become a buddha during my pregnancy with Jackson; I became Rambo. I strapped on my ammunition, my night-vision goggles, and popped a few grenades in my pockets and set off into a jungle of terror. It came down to a simple cost-benefit analysis. I knew that I wanted a baby so badly that I would risk the devastating disappointment of another loss.

Just last week, I spoke to a woman who had suffered two very late miscarriages in a row. She was still reeling from her most recent loss and was asking me that same heartbreaking question: How am I going to have the courage to do this again? So I shared with her my Rambo story.

"Are you sure you're my yoga teacher?" she asked.

"Yes. I'm teaching you Rambo Fertility Yoga," I replied.

So here's what I told her. Literally imagine that you are a fearless person—whether that's Rambo (my image) or Joan of Arc or a Resistance fighter during World War II—and each morning put on all your trappings of fearlessness. Whether it's Rambo's Uzi or fishnet stockings with a pistol tucked into your garter, or a suit of shining armor, put it on. When the waves of panic start to roll in you can rest your hand on your sword hilt. It's amazing how brave you can become when call on these archetypes of courage.

While it may sound silly, using this sort of visualization to conquer a fear can be enormously cleansing. By choosing an archetype of courage we become courageous ourselves. The fear and panic thoughts that arise have no place to stick to this image and, with effort and conviction, they become just that—thoughts.

Welcoming Your Past

The first step in the mental cleansing of toxic memories is to acknowledge them. It is important to just welcome in your experiences and memories as they are rather than trying to repress or avert them. The key word here is "welcome." We didn't say you have to like your past; just welcome it for what it is. If it was painful or emotional, just acknowledge that it was painful or emotional. Don't attach to these feelings; just watch and welcome them.

Often, we hold onto our toxic experiences and adjust our future actions accordingly. Sometimes our actions are completely unconscious. We're not exactly sure why we feel anxious or stressed about a situation; we just do. There are many examples of this at Pulling Down the Moon. Think about the woman who has experienced multiple miscarriages. Each and every one of those miscarriages can shape her future attitudes about herself, her partner, and her fertility. Her miscarriage becomes her story and she attaches to it as a way to further define who she is.

Sometimes we become so connected to our stories that we cannot break away from the feelings and fear they evoke. We worry that our stories will always have the same tragic ending and, as a result, fear becomes so intense that pregnancy, when it does happen, becomes a completely stressful and agonizing experience. It may be impossible to change our past, but it is possible to go back and reconstruct our erroneous beliefs, attitudes, and thoughts about that event. One way to do this is to stop defining ourselves by our stories and stop believing the ending will always be the same.

SYMBOLS AND WHY THEY ARE IMPORTANT

Symbols pervade our world, whether we are aware of them or not. We choose to drive a Porsche because Porsche has lead us to believe that their car is the symbol of prosperity and prestige. We drive a hybrid car because it is the symbol of environmental conservation. We choose our clothes based on how a designer markets them and how the clothes, in turn, make us feel when we wear them. We say with pride we are wearing the status symbol of Chanel, Dolce & Gabbana, Guess or Calvin Klein. If we presented you with a piece of paper that contained only a big red bulls-eye would you know the symbol? How about the symbol of yellow arches?

Sometimes we don't even need to explain what the symbol is. We just recognize the yellow arches as McDonald's, and the symbol alone may trigger a very physiological reaction in the mind or body. It may stir up childhood memories of enjoying a Shamrock shake with Mom and Dad before the St. Patrick's Day Parade. Maybe it calls to mind a favorite teenage meeting place after your high school football games. The symbol may create a physical effect in the body, such as a grumbling stomach or the mouth watering for a Big Mac. Crazier still, the symbol might create an emotion inside you—perhaps anger that our society has become less nutrition conscious or anxiety because you worry about how your craving for that Big Mac might affect your fertility.

Beyond the car you drive and the clothes you wear, have you ever wondered what other symbols have made their way into your home? How about the artwork on your walls? Are they pictures of faraway beaches and palm trees, or maybe animals running free in the wild? Why did you put them there? And what do they symbolize to you? People attach to certain symbols to explain who they are or where they are going. There are some symbols that are very powerful and can tell an entire story just by us looking at them. Think about the crucifix, the star of David, or the swastika.

A Radical Thought

Symbolists believe that every symbol from every religion can be read esoterically. While each of the glyphs and symbols might be different, it is believed that if you break down each of the more complex symbols into their simplest form, they are largely the same. Think about the Christian cross which is really a four-pointed star. A star is also seen in Judaism and a star and crescent symbolize Islam. If we were to use the intelligence of ancient symbolism to interpret the relationship between these three religions, we might conclude that while each is somewhat different (4-points, 6-points and 5-points + crescent), the basic symbol is the same (the star). We might then intuit that all three may have beliefs in common. In our simplest form, we are all one.

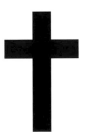 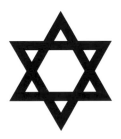 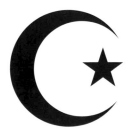

What's a Symbol

So what exactly is a symbol? By definition, a symbol is a pictorial expression of an idea or thought. The earliest writing had no characters; instead, symbols stood for an entire sentence or a whole phrase. Think of hieroglyphics and the picture writings of the cave man. In essence, a symbol is a parable, and a parable is a spoken symbol.

Psychologists, yogis, and sages alike agree that symbols can be important in raising our consciousness because they convey something more than the obvious. The psychologist might show you a series of ink blots and ask you what they mean. The yogi might ask you to meditate on how your physical yoga practice is a symbol for how you approach life. For instance, if you get frustrated because you can't put your foot behind your head and push yourself to a point of discomfort, is that symbolic of how you approach other challenges in your life: you push to the point of pain and agitation?

You might be wondering how this concept of symbolism ever got started. It is believed that prophets and seers from thousands of years ago needed a way to record their insights and then teach their followers. They knew that their followers could not possibly retain everything they were taught in their memories, so they came up with geometric shapes and glyphs as a way to help them remember. Before the seer accepted her beliefs to be true, she would test them through her own spiritual visions and then verify her concepts with other wise seers and prophets. Nothing was accepted as correct thinking unless it agreed with the research and experiences of other adepts.

These symbols were also important because they characterized those things that were above scientific reasoning and beyond the intellect. Remember: These were the visions of the wisest of people. Creating a symbol was an attempt to tap into Awareness. It was believed that if the symbol was not able to transcend the thinking brain and be understood at a deeper level, the concept would fade-out from human remembrance.

A Note about Awareness

We don't capitalize the word Awareness to be cute. Awareness is not a state; it simply is. We don't have to achieve anything to experience it because it is our birthright. It exists without beginning or end and permeates every fiber of our being, whether we can see it or not. If we cannot see it, it is because we are attached to thought patterns and emotions that we are allowing to create our world or define our life. When we begin to recognize these thoughts and patterns, we do so from a point of Awareness. When we step into this space of Awareness, it is radiant, spacious, peaceful—and it is bliss.

Symbols as Patterns in our World

The ancient sages also discovered that many symbols could be found over and over again in nature. Many referred to them as sacred geometry because they seem to be the very building blocks that create the architecture of our physical world. They believed that tapping into these symbols or geometric shapes could help us understand how things are interrelated and how all things are really different manifestations of the same symbols, such as the star, the square, and the triangle.

The sages also believed that when you start using these symbols to build something, similar patterns would emerge over and over again and the same basic geometric shapes could be found within the patterns. Within these patterns, there also appeared to be mathematical relationships and constants occurring again and again, such as the Golden Ratio of 1.6180339887… which is present throughout nature, as in the florets of a pine cone, for example.

Using Symbols to Understand Your Thoughts

The ancients also believed that the study of symbols could be important as we try to make sense of seemingly nonsensical thoughts, patterns, or events in our lives. In a very practical way, the study of our own symbols can be useful in trying to understand a powerful dream that we had, a pattern in our lives that we can't break, or even an irrational fear. All this may sound like very hard work for the purposes of a cleanse program, but at the very least, the study of symbols is a great exercise for the mind.

Working with symbols also helps develop our intuition. This is a really important part of the infertility cleanse because our thinking brains can hold us hostage to irrational thoughts and emotions that often make us feel like we are crazy people. Our thoughts can create stress in mind and body, which can lead to toxicity and dis-ease; therefore, developing our intuition can be an important tool in helping us understand the origin of a thought.

So we've looked a bit at modern-day symbols and got a bit of a history lesson on the origin of the symbols of old. The next step is to learn how to take the wisdom of ancient symbols and apply it to the present. In other words, how do we make the understanding of symbols practical for today and for our Cleanse Lifestyle?

Perhaps the following real-life story about the power of symbols will shed some light. Lady Chatterly's Story:

The "Fertility Clinic" Symbol

We had a patient come to Pulling Down the Moon who was in her early 40s, had been trying to get pregnant for years, but had a complete aversion to medical fertility treatment. She did acupuncture, yoga, reiki, and sought spiritual guidance at Pulling Down the Moon. Even though she felt better and calmer, she wasn't getting pregnant. We asked her to use the symbols in her dreams and to meditate more fully on where the aversion to medical treatment may have come from. She came to us after she had her own "aha" moment.

She learned from her own hard work that she was avoiding seeing a fertility doctor because it had become for her a symbol of some sort of short-coming or failure. She couldn't bear to feel any more self-loathing. In time, she saw that her feelings were just irrational thoughts floating around in her head. She learned to recognize these thoughts and just welcome them without judgment. In fact, she even gave a name to these incessant thoughts and personified them by referring to them as Lady Chatterly.

She learned to laugh at the dialogue going on in her head and eventually sought medical treatment for her infertility. Over time, she decided it was most important for her to just be a parent and it really mattered less how that baby would come to her. She opened her heart to donor eggs and has since delivered a healthy baby. Once she held that baby in her arms, her fertility story that she connected with for so many years just somehow faded away as did the power of the symbol.

In fact, the symbol now had become just the opposite. It now represented triumph and fertility, both literally and emotionally.

Lifestyle Cleansing: Putting It All Together

In **SECTION 1** of this book, we took a very scientific look at how the body processes toxins and what kinds of toxicity exists in our world today. **SECTION 2** straddled both medical science and mysticism in understanding how the mind can work as an organ of detox by helping us connect more fully with Awareness and by becoming less attached emotionally to our stories from the past.

SECTION 3 is designed to be a synthesis of these two prior sections. It provides a practical way for you to create a successful home-based Lifestyle Cleanse that is safe and specifically designed for women trying to conceive. Some of these processes are simple or ritualistic in nature and can be explained in one page. Others require more in-depth study. It is our hope that each of the processes we recommend in this Lifestyle section helps you gain greater insight into yourself as a whole person.

While doing each exercise in this section ask yourself the following two questions:
1. How does any one activity or exercise make me feel?
2. What have I learned about myself, and how can I take these insights and apply them to my life to find greater health and well-being?

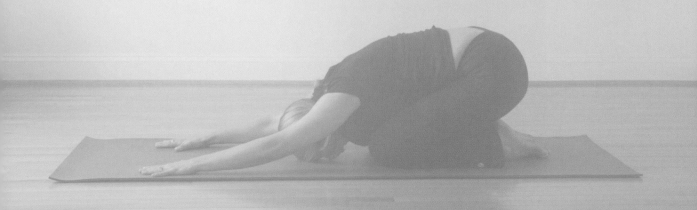

CHAPTER 8

The Cleansing Power of Food

In this chapter, we will synthesize all the information we have provided thus far into easy-to-follow guidelines for eating that supports optimal fertility and limits exposure to both endogenous (coming from you) and exogenous (coming from the environment) toxicity. You may be surprised that putting together an eating plan that supports optimal health and fertility isn't a raw-food or a wheat grass endeavor. Our goal, instead, is to create a nutritious and satisfying eating program that:

1. Limits fertility "no" foods like refined sugar and carbs, food additives like hormones, pesticides, and artificial colors/flavors, excess caffeine, and alcohol.
2. Balances blood sugar levels.
3. Limits inflammation and oxidative stress and feeds your body's innate ability to maintain healthy tissues.
4. Supports gut health.
5. Helps the liver do what it is supposed to do: eliminate substances that should not be allowed to build up in the body.

Prep Time: Out With the Old!

Before beginning this program, we recommend you spend three days reading labels and getting a handle on what you are really eating. You may be surprised to learn that you're doing better than you thought… or you may find that when you're honest with yourself you probably could be eating a lot better. If you discover you fall into the latter category, don't become discouraged; be happy—you may have the most to gain by making the changes outlined in this chapter! As you move through this program, you will likely find yourself making many changes quite naturally as a result of this new awareness.

At the end of this chapter you will find our Baseline Worksheet. The Baseline Worksheet includes a seven-day grid, with space on each day to record what you eat for breakfast, lunch, dinner, and snacks. At the end of each day, and using the GO/WHOA/NO worksheet as your guide, take a green highlighter and highlight all the fertility "go" foods you ate in green, highlight fertility "whoa" foods in yellow, and fertility "no" in pink. While you may have a worksheet that looks like a rainbow now, in a few weeks your goal is to have a primarily green—GO!—page with a sprinkling of sunshine yellow.

Record everything—and read every label. You will learn a lot about the foods you are currently eating, and you will also feel a tremendous sense of accomplishment when, in time, you can look back and see how far you've come!

General Fertility Nutrition Guidelines

Eat a diet with "high nutrient density," or, put more simply, get as many vitamins and minerals per calorie as you can from the food you eat. A piece of candy and a carrot stick have roughly the same amount of calories. Which do you think is more nutrient dense?

1. Eat fertility-smart carbohydrates. Low-glycemic, high-fiber carbohydrates are key to a fertility-friendly diet. When reading your labels, avoid simple carbohydrates (sugars, high-fructose corn syrup, highly refined grains, etc.).
2. Choose healthy fats. Diets high in saturated and trans fats are associated with higher rates of ovulatory infertility. Increase your intake of monounsaturated and omega-3 polyunsaturated fats. Read labels. Avoid hydrogenated fats and partially hydrogenated fats.
3. Eat adequate amounts of lean protein from hormone- and contaminant-free sources.

4. Go big "O." Eat organic, whenever possible. Pesticides and chemicals used in conventional farming can disrupt hormone function.
5. Eat a minimum of one serving of the following fertility-friendly foods each day: lentils/beans, cruciferous vegetables, and healthy fats (olive oil, avocado, approved fish).

6. Eat a warming diet (see below).

Warming Diet

Both Ayurveda (the traditional Indian medicine of which yoga is part) and TCM recommend that women who are trying to conceive limit cold and raw foods. The rationale behind this recommendation is that cold or raw foods require extra energy to digest, which draws energy away from the other organ systems. This recommendation can be challenging, as we are encourage women to eat more fruits and vegetables and certainly don't want to discourage this practice. If, however, you're someone who eats a salad at every meal with a cold soda and some frozen yogurt on the side, this recommendation is for you. On the other hand, if you struggle to eat vegetables and only like them crunchy and raw, by all means eating them that way is better than not eating them at all. At Pulling Down the Moon, we believe the optimal diet for fertility is a warming diet, and while we do not forbid patients from eating a salad or crudités, we encourage the following practices:

1. Substitute warming foods for cooling foods. For example, try vegetable soup or a stir-fry instead of salad.
2. Limit raw and cold (temperature) foods and beverages.
3. When you do choose salad, consume a warming drink along side.
4. Increase warming methods of preparation that preserve the nutritional quality of food (bake, stir-fry, and sauté rather than boil or fry).
5. When possible allow chilled foods to reach room temperature before eating.

FERTILITY GO, WHOA, AND NO FOODS

The box below gives a general idea of serving sizes for most food groups. Because determining your personal caloric requirement is beyond the scope of this book, we recommend you use this information as a guideline when speaking to your nutritionist about a personalized eating plan.

Food Groups	One Serving Size Equals...
Breads, Cereals, Rice, Pasta, and other Grains	- 1 slice bread or ½ bagel the size of a hockey puck. - ½-cup cooked rice or pasta would fill a cupcake wrapper.
Fruits and Vegetables	- One fruit and vegetable serving is equal to a piece the size of a tennis ball. A ½-cup of cut fruit would fill a cupcake wrapper.
Meat, Chicken, Fish, Dry Beans and Peas, Eggs, and Nuts	- 3 ounces lean meat, chicken, or fish is approximately the same size as a deck of cards or a check book. - A good rule of thumb is to use the palm of your hand to measure meat and poultry, while your whole hand represents a serving of fish.
Dairy	- 1 ounce cheese equals about 4 dice
Fats, Oils, and Sweets	- Use sparingly. One teaspoon of fat is equal to the end of your thumb, from the knuckle up.

Here is a simple guide to foods that we consider to be Fertility GO Foods, Fertility WHOA Foods, and Fertility NO Foods. You will use this list to evaluate your current diet and to build your optimal one.

FERTILITY GO FOODS

GO foods are things that you should go out of your way to eat every day. They contain the nutrients that support fertility and, in some cases, have very specific roles to play in your reproductive health. We recommend that as far as budget allows you choose organic/transitional fruits and vegetables and grass/wild-fed meats raised without hormones.

1. Antioxidant-Rich Fruits/Vegetables

Servings: 1-2 per day
- Berries
- Dark leafy green vegetables
- Dark orange, yellow and green vegetables like squash, tomatoes, red and green peppers, and broccoli

Fertility Connection: Almost all veggies and fruit contain one of more of the antioxidant compounds vitamin C, selenium, and beta carotene. These compounds help to "quench" potential oxidative damage by Reactive Oxygen Species (ROS) and tip the balance away from oxidative stress and toward good antioxidant status.

2. Cruciferous Vegetables

Servings: 1-2 per day
- Cabbage, broccoli, cauliflower, Brussels sprouts, kale and collard greens (technically these last two are Brassica vegetables).

Fertility Connection: These veggies contain a compound called indole-3-carbinol (I-3-C for short) that regulates estrogen metabolism and helps convert "bad estrogens" into good ones.

THE BEST VEGGIES EVER!

There's no getting around the fact that a fertility-friendly diet is rich in fruits and vegetables. From the perspective of traditional medical sciences like Oriental Medicine and Ayurveda, the fertility diet should also be warming, which means that very little raw food should be consumed. This can be a real challenge for those of us who love raw veggies and eat two salads a day. Fear not, friends, here are some unbelievably delicious ways to cook vegetables, not just to preserve nutrients, but to taste great as well!

Asparagus

- Trust us that this is the absolutely easiest and most delicious way to eat asparagus.
- Trim tough ends from stalks.
- Toss with 1 T olive oil on a baking sheet and broil for 7-8 minutes, shaking pan one time during this process.
- Finish with a sprinkle of kosher salt and a squeeze of lime juice if you wish.

Green Beans

- Line baking sheet with foil and preheat oven to 400 degrees F.
- Toss beans with 1 T olive oil and roast for 20-25 minutes, turning once to promote even browning.

Green Peas

Did you know that when petite pois (small green peas) first came to the court of Louis XIV at Versailles, they were considered the greatest of delicacies and served for dessert? Thanks to Cook's Illustrated Magazine for this ingenious and delicious way to cook frozen peas.

- Add frozen peas directly to a pan with sautéed aromatics (garlic or shallots cooked in olive oil until they smell good).
- Cover to capture the steam and warm the peas through.
- For special occasions or when company comes, try adding a teaspoon of sugar per pound of peas to spruce up the flavor even more.

Broccoli - for 1 ¾ pounds

- Pan-roasting broccoli emphasizes its sweetness and disguises the sulfurous flavors of cruciferous vegetables.
- Prior to cooking, cut florets into 1 ½-inch pieces. You can use the stalk, too. Just shave off the outer 1/8-inch of stalk and then slice on the bias into 1 ½-inch pieces.
- Film a nonstick* skillet with a generous tablespoon of olive oil, add the stalks, and cook for 2 minutes. To promote browning (yummy sweetness!), cook on medium heat and do not stir. Add florets and cook until they start to brown (1-2 minutes) and then add 3T water, cover and cook for 2 minutes.
- Remove lid and cook until water is gone and broccoli is tender (about 2 more minutes).

Cauliflower - for 1 head

- Preheat oven to 475 degrees F.
- Trim leaves, cut cauliflower into large wedges, toss with olive oil, and roast on a foil-lined baking sheet and cover with foil.
- Roast covered for the first 10 minutes, then remove foil and cook for an additional 15-20 minutes, flipping wedges once to promote browning.

Carrots

You won't believe how sweet and delicious carrots can be!

- Peel and slice carrots into thin rounds (using the food processor is a quick way to do this).
- Heat olive oil in a heavy skillet and add carrots.
- Sauté on medium heat without stirring for about 3-5 minutes to promote browning.
- Stir and cook for 3-5 minutes more.
- For added flavor, drizzle good balsamic vinegar over the carrots when you first add them to the pan.
- Finish with fresh ground black pepper and a sprinkle of kosher salt.

Zucchini

Okay, so this veggie can be challenging. Too many seeds and a delicate flavor turn to mush even with a sauté pan and the best of intentions. Again, Cook's Illustrated saves the day:

- Choose zucchini smaller than 1 inch in diameter for more flavor and less water.
- Cut into 3-inch chunks and then shred on the large holes of a box grater, rotating the piece as needed to shred the meat but avoid the seeds and core (which you can discard!).
- Place zucchini in a colander, salt (about 1 ½ teaspoons for 2 ½ pounds of zucchini) and let sit for 10 minutes.
- Place shredded squash in a kitchen towel and wring out excess moisture. Do this in batches, so you can really get the wetness out.
- Toss the dried zucchini with a teaspoon or two of olive oil and then cook lightly in a non-stick skillet filmed with about 2 more teaspoons of olive oil.
- Cook over medium heat for about 4 minutes, stirring frequently to promote browning.

* A note about non-stick cookware. Non-stick pans can be an important part of healthy cooking and eating because they allow us to cut down on the amount of fat we need to use. In recent years, however, there has been valid concern that non-stick pans are a significant source of toxic exposure to perfluorooctanoic acid (PFOA), a likely carcinogen. Subsequent study has shown that non-stick pans can release this substance as a gas when heated to very high temperatures. To ensure safe usage of your non-stick, don't leave your pans unattended on the flame, don't preheat an empty pan, do not use higher than a medium flame with your non-stick and experiment with other cookware, including cast iron and steel.

3. Assorted Whole Grains

- Servings: 2-3 per day
- Barley, millet, brown rice, amaranth, quinoa, oats
- For a real nutrition boost, limit your wheat intake to one wheat product per day, and explore other whole grains (see text box) and whole grain flours.

Fertility Connection: Whole grains are an excellent source of B vitamins and fiber. For optimal gut health, experiment with many different grains. We recommend a wide range of grains since many women largely limit their whole grain intake to wheat. Wheat is on the list of "top offenders" when it comes to food sensitivity.

ADVENTURES IN FERTILITY-FRIENDLY EATING: A WHOLE (GRAIN) NEW WORLD

Spelt

Spelt is a high-protein ancient grain that is generally ground into flour. Spelt's tough outer husk may actually protect the nutrient content when it is ground into flour. The flavor of spelt is nuttier and sweeter than wheat. Spelt has gluten, just like wheat, so it is not suitable for a gluten-free diet. Some individuals who are sensitive to wheat may be able to tolerate spelt, perhaps because it's an ancient form of wheat and has been part of the human food supply for so long.

Barley

Barley is a fabulous fertility grain. While it does contain some gluten (5-8 percent of protein) and may not be suitable for a gluten-free diet it does have many other good qualities. Barley is an excellent source of fiber, particularly beta-glucan soluble fiber, which has been shown to slow glucose absorption. Barley is also unique in that, in contrast to most other grains that contain fiber only in the outer bran, it contains fiber throughout the entire kernel. Barley flakes can be cooked and eaten for breakfast or ground into flour and used in baked goods.

Barley for Breakfast

- 2/3-cup water
- 1/3-cup barley flakes
- Pinch salt, optional
- Optional additions: chopped banana, dried cranberries or blueberries, chopped walnuts, drizzle of agave nectar
- In 4-cup microwave-proof container, combine water, barley, salt, and fruit of choice. Microwave on HIGH power for 3 minutes. Stir. Continue to microwave on HIGH power for 3 minutes longer. Cool slightly and serve. Makes 1 serving.

Millet

Millet is thought to be one of the first grains cultivated by humans. It is gluten-free and slightly higher in fat than wheat, although the fat is largely unsaturated and contains more omega-3 fatty acids than other grains. Millet can be cooked "pilaf style" or used ground, as in millet flour. Millet is a mild thyroid peroxidase inhibitor, so individuals with thyroid disease should not consumer millet in large quantities.

Fluffy Cooked Millet

- Toast 1 cup millet first by adding grain to a dry pot and stirring constantly over medium heat for 3-4 minutes until a nutty aroma begins to arise. Once millet begins to "pop," add 2 cups of veggie stock or boiling water and return to a boil.
- Reduce heat, cover, and simmer 20-25 minutes, or until liquid has been absorbed. Remove from heat and allow to rest for 5 minutes covered. Fluff and serve. For a moister, more risotto-esque millet use 3 cups of liquid.

Quinoa

Quinoa is a gluten-free grain that is high in protein—about 18 percent of quinoa calories come from protein. Moreover, unlike wheat and rice, which lack the amino acid lysine, quinoa is a complete protein. Quinoa must be soaked to remove the saponins, bitter-tasting chemicals that can be found on the surface of the grain.

Basic Quinoa

- Bring two cups water and one cup pre-soaked quinoa to a boil in a sauce pan and cook, covered, at a low simmer for 15-18 minutes. Use vegetable or chicken stock to add flavor. Serve with bitter greens, like kale or collards, or with diced tomatoes and fresh herbs.

Amaranth

Another gluten-free grain, amaranth is a rock star when it comes to protein—one serving of amaranth can provide 60 percent of daily iron needs. This grain is an excellent source of the sulfur-containing amino acid methionine. Traditionally, amaranth is considered a "healing" grain, the perfect food for those on the mend from illness. Like millet, amaranth has a good amount of oil, about 6-10 percent by volume, including tocotrienols (a form of vitamin E) and linolenic acid (an omega-3 PUFA). Amaranth has a sticky texture, as opposed to "fluffier" grains like quinoa and rice. It can also be popped like popcorn and added for crunch to other dishes.

Basic Amaranth

- 2.5 cups liquid
- 1 cup amaranth seeds
- Simmer for 20 minutes, or until seeds are tender and somewhat sticky.

Sweet Amaranth

- Substitute apple juice for water, and add cinnamon or ginger.

Savory Amaranth

- Substitute chicken/vegetable stock for water and finish with fresh herbs, a toss of olive oil, and a sprinkle of salt.

4. Healthy Fats

- Servings: 2-3 per day
- Olive oil
- Nut oils (such as walnut oil)
- Dark leafy greens (trace amounts)
- Nuts

Fertility Connection: The fats we eat play a very important role in fertility. They are incorporated into our cell membranes (think egg and sperm) and are the key constituent in many important molecules in our body, including hormones. Monounsaturated fats help to lower levels of harmful LDL ("bad") cholesterol and are found in olive oil, avocado and most nuts. Monounsaturated fats may also play a role in lowering inflammation. Omega-3 fats are key to lowering the level of inflammation in our body and are found in fatty cold-water fish, dark leafy vegetables, walnuts, chia, and flax seeds. Healthy fats make for healthy cells and reduce inflammation. Because fatty fish are one of the foods we must limit in the fertility-friendly diet, we recommend that women who are trying to conceive supplement with a high-quality fish oil supplement.

HEALTHY FATS VS. UNHEALTHY FATS

Healthy Fats	Food Sources
Monounsaturated Fat	olive oil, peanut oil, canola oil, avocados, nuts, and seeds
Omega-3 fatty acids	Fatty cold-water fish (wild salmon, mackerel, and herring), flax seeds, flax seed oil, and walnuts
Fats to Limit	**Food Sources**
Omega-6 fatty acids	Vegetable oils (safflower, sunflower, corn, soybean)
Saturated fats	Animal fats, including those found in meat, poultry, eggs, dairy, lard, butter, and coconut oil, as well as palm oil. Grass-fed meat will have a significantly healthier fat composition than grain-fed meat.
Unhealthy Fats	**Food Sources**
Trans fat	Partially hydrogenated vegetable oils, fried foods, shortening, and margarine

5. Lean Protein

Servings: 2-3 per day

- Free-range poultry
- Grass-fed beef
- Exotic game meats, including bison, ostrich, and venison
- Free-range organic eggs

Fertility Connection: Protein is important for the creation and repair of body tissues, and the amino acid building blocks of protein play a major role in our body's detoxification processes. Choose lean proteins like free-range organic chicken and turkey and free-range organic eggs. Experiment with exotic game meats like bison, ostrich, or venison.

6. Beans and Lentils

- Servings: 1 per day

Fertility Connection: At least one serving of protein per day should come from a vegetarian source, such as lentils, black beans, chick peas, and other nutritionally dense legumes and pulses. Besides being a good source of protein, beans and lentils contain soluble fiber, which helps bind excess hormones and remove them from the body. The undigested remnants of fiber from beans and lentils are one of the favorite foods of "good" bacteria in the gut.

7. Lignins

- Servings: 1-2 per day, most likely in your fruit, vegetables, and lentils already
- Good sources of lignins are fruit with edible seeds (berries), root vegetables and beans. Seeds such as flax and chia are also rich in lignins.

Fertility Connection: Lignins are a form of soluble fiber and serve a myriad of purposes in the body. Lignins are another favorite food of beneficial bacteria and help to speed food through the digestive system. Lignins have also been shown to inhibit the action of aromatase, the enzyme that converts fat to estrogen in breast and adipose tissue.

Cleansing Tip: Aromatase Inhibition

Only in recent years has our understanding of the complex relationship between diet and hormone health deepened to the point where we can definitively say that what we eat affects our hormone function. Much of this understanding has come from research into estrogen-related cancers like breast cancer. Excitingly, much of this information can be applied in theory and practice to the world of infertility. One such case is the enzyme aromatase.

AROMATASE is the enzyme produced in breast and fat cells that converts the weak androgens androstenedione and testosterone into estrogen. As a result, excess aromatase activity can increase estrogen production and potentially disrupt normal reproductive function. This is important from a dietary standpoint as some food compounds inhibit aromatase activity. Foods that limit aromatase activity include:

LIGNINS: lignins are soluble fiber and are converted to the "mammalian lignins" enterodiol and enterlacton by intestinal bacteria. These compounds inhibit aromatase activity and may also act as estrogen inhibitors in the body. Lignins are also one of the favorite foods of beneficial bacteria in our gut and help to speed food through the digestive system. Good sources of lignins are: fruit with edible seeds (berries), root vegetables, flax, and chia seeds.

FLAVANOIDS like quercetin (found in onions, cabbage, garlic, apples, and berries), apigenin (celery, parsley, basil, artichokes, and chamomile), narigenin (citrus fruit), resveratrol (red wine and grapes) and oleuopein (olive oil). (Adlerkreutz et al, 2007)

FERTILITY WHOA FOODS

WHOA foods are foods that should stop you in your tracks before eating them. They should be eaten sparingly, a maximum of one serving daily.

1. Fish

Unfortunately, due to stresses on the environment, the healthy protein found in fish must be consumed with care.

- **HIGHEST MERCURY** (AVOID EATING): Grouper, marlin, orange roughy, tilefish, swordfish, shark, mackerel (king).

- **HIGH MERCURY** (Eat no more than three 6-oz servings per month): Bass (saltwater), croaker, halibut, tuna (canned, white albacore), tuna (fresh bluefin, ahi), sea trout, bluefish, lobster (American/Maine).
- **LOWER MERCURY** (Eat no more than six 6-oz servings per month): Carp, mahi mahi, crab (Dungeness), snapper, crab (blue), herring, crab (snow), monkfish, perch (freshwater), skate, cod, tuna (canned, chunk light), tuna (fresh Pacific albacore).
- **LOWEST MERCURY** (Enjoy two 6-oz servings per week): Anchovies, butterfish, calamari (squid), caviar (farmed), crab (king), pollock, catfish, whitefish, perch (ocean), scallops, flounder, haddock, hake, herring, lobster (spiny/rock), shad, sole, crawfish/crayfish, salmon, shrimp, clams, tilapia, oysters, sardines, sturgeon (farmed), trout (freshwater). (Data obtained from the Natural Resource Defense Council (NRDC), the FDA, and the EPA.)

In addition to choosing low-risk fish, we also recommend that for the health of the planet you choose sustainable, wild-caught fish. Choosing wild-caught over farmed fish may also confer health benefits as farmed fish have been shown to have higher levels of some pesticides and PCBs and may have lower levels of healthy fats than wild caught counterparts.

2. Fermented Soy
- Tofu
- Tempeh

There is evidence that soy intake in men is associated with sub-fertility and, while still controversial, data in women suggests that the estrogenic compounds in soy may lengthen or disrupt the menstrual cycle. Apart from hormonal concerns, soy is one of the most common food intolerances. We recommend the consumption of fermented soy foods (tofu and tempeh) over processed soy foods (textured vegetable protein (TVP) and other soy meat replacements that fracture soy into isolated soy proteins) because fermented soy is easier to digest. Soy should be eaten sparingly—no more than one 8 oz serving per day.

3. Dairy
When it comes to fertility, we have some important information to share with you about dairy foods. The Nurses Study 2 data indicates that one serving of full-fat dairy per day is associated with a lower risk of ovulatory infertility (OI), while intake of low-fat dairy is linked to higher rates of OI. Yes, you read that right: full-fat dairy is better for you. Apart from being a potentially allergenic food, by its nature milk contains not only added growth hormones contributed by agribusiness but also the reproductive hormones of the cows themselves. In modern dairies, it is

common practice to milk pregnant cows, which have very high levels of estrogen circulating in their milk. In response to increasing evidence that low-fat milk, factory-farmed milk may not be the healthy food we once believed, there has been a trend toward the consumption of raw milk in recent years. While advocates swear by the safety of these products there have been outbreaks of food-borne illness in past years that relate back to the consumption of raw dairy. In our opinion, raw milk products should be avoided, especially during pregnancy until the testing and safety of such products are better established. More interesting in our opinion is the technique of low-temperature, small batch pasteurization that is currently gaining ground in small micro-dairies. Small batch milk is generally cream-top (non-homogenized) which advocates claim promote better absorption of the nutrients in the milk and preserve enzymes in the milk that aid digestion. Look for pasture-fed cows as well. Grass-fed animals produce milk that is higher in CLA (conjugated linoleic acids) a healthy form of fat that may prevent cancer. We recommend you do not consume more than one 8 oz serving of dairy per day and choose full-fat dairy over lower fat.

FERTILITY NO FOODS

1. Refined Sugars

Refined sugars have only a small place in the fertility diet. In general, our recommendation is to limit the intake of refined sugar to less than 5 percent of total calories (so, if you're eating a 2000-calorie diet, no more than 100 calories of sugar each day). This includes white and brown sugar, honey, and other caloric sweeteners. This does not mean you must lead a treat-free existence. We recommend you use your 100 "sweet" calories toward something very yummy, like a square of dark chocolate or a coconut frozen fruit bar (with a cup of tea of course!). Here's a hint - one gram of sugar (or any carb) has 4 calories. Read labels and make educated decisions. One serving of 72% cocoa dark chocolate (about 43 g) contains just 11 grams of refined sugars - and 4 g of dietary fiber. Remember, though, that many processed foods contain surprisingly high levels of refined sugars - so read labels and don't blow your sweet budget on ketchup!

2. Sugar Substitutes

Sugar substitutes are not part of a fertility-friendly diet. Studies suggest that intake of non-caloric sugar substitutes can actually lead to subsequent overeating. Many non-caloric sweeteners contain chemicals whose actions in the body are not well understood. Two sugar substitutes that are permissible in very limited amounts in a fertility-friendly diet are stevia and agave nectar. Please note that agave nectar, not technically a sugar-substitute, is not non-caloric. Again, the idea is to heal our sweet tooth. Use all sweeteners, natural and artificial, sparingly.

3. Refined Carbohydrates

Bye-bye white bread and other processed grains. If it's not whole grain, it's not on the table. And as we mentioned above: there are many other grains besides wheat we can use as substitutes whole grains.

4. Inflammation-Promoting Foods

Red meat, trans fat, highly processed carbohydrates and sugars promote inflammation. Limit these foods in your diet.

RECOMMENDATIONS FOR ANTI-INFLAMMATORY EATING

The typical Western diet is filled with foods that promote an inflammatory environment in the body, so our diet is one area where we can actively combat chronic inflammation that leads to modern diseases and fertility problems.

Foods to be Avoided

Foods that feed the fire of inflammation and should be avoided include:

- Polyunsaturated cheap vegetable oils high in omega-6 fatty acids (Safflower, sunflower, corn, peanut and soy). Omega-6 fatty acids are easily converted to arachadonic acid, which has a highly pro-inflammatory action in the body.

- High-glycemic carbohydrates ("fast" carbs) raise blood sugar and stimulate higher levels of insulin than low-glycemic (slow-burning) carbohydrates. Insulin stimulates the action of inflammatory chemicals and prompts enzymes to release arachidonic acid into the blood.

- Saturated fat in high-fat factory-farmed dairy and red meat contain arachidonic acid and can increase levels of pro-inflammatory chemicals in the body. In addition, most commercially produced livestock are fed an almost exclusively corn diet, resulting in meat with high concentrations of omega-6 fats.

- Trans fats found in highly processed foods also exacerbate the inflammation response and are associated with higher levels of ovulatory infertility. Experts theorize that our high consumption of man-made trans fats (they're everywhere in our processed-foods world) create an environment where trans fats are becoming integrated into key fatty components in the body, such as cell membranes and our fat cells.
  Trans fats also stimulate the production of LDL ("bad") cholesterol, which causes inflammation in our blood vessels (as opposed to HDL cholesterol, which is good for us). It's even possible that trans fats contribute to hormonal dysfunction and insulin resistance. Receptors for our reproductive hormones perch in the phospholipid bilayer that forms the cell membrane. If trans fats infiltrate this important barrier, cells may become less efficient in their ability to send and receive hormonal signals.
  Look for products that indicate they are "trans fat-free," and completely avoid all trans fats when you're trying to conceive. Remember, it may not say, "trans fat" on the food label. Look for "partially hydrogenated oils" (these are vegetable oils that have been made solid at room temperature by the addition of hydrogen (hydrogenated) during manufacturing).

> **Foods that reduce Inflammation**
>
> On the other hand, there are foods that are known to halt inflammation:
>
> – Fruits and vegetables contain substances that can reduce inflammation.
> – Healthy fats like monounsaturated olive and canola oil and omega-3 essential fatty acids can serve as very powerful anti-inflammatory agents. Omega-3 fatty acids are found in cold-water oily fish, walnuts, flax seeds, canola oil, and pumpkin seeds.
> – Lean protein from fish, game, and chicken that have spent their lives foraging for food. Limit red meat intake, except for bison and venison or other game meats. Game meats and free-range pastured poultry have meat that is much higher in omega-3 fatty acids than the corn-fed meat of factory farmed animals. The same is true for range pastured eggs and milk from pasture-fed cows which can be a truly rich source of healthy omega-3 fats.
> – Fiber has been shown to reduce one major marker of inflammation, C-Reactive Protein (CRP).

5. Trans Fats

- Read labels
- Found in margarine, processed foods, and baked goods

Trans fats should be completely eliminated from the diet. They are associated with higher rates of ovulatory infertility, inflammation, and poor egg and sperm quality.

6. Alcohol

Most studies suggest that alcohol intake is deleterious for fertility. However, at least one study has shown that wine drinkers got pregnant quicker than abstainers or the consumers of other alcoholic beverages. Because of the evidence that intake of alcoholic beverages is associated with higher levels of oxidative stress, we recommend that alcohol consumption is limited to 1-2 glasses of red wine per week and eliminated one month prior to starting an ART cycle.

7. Caffeine

Caffeine should be limited to less than 50 mg/day, or ideally, eliminated. To put this in context, a grande cup of coffee from Starbucks contains roughly 330 mg of caffeine.

FOOD AND MOOD

Depression, as you likely know, is linked to higher rates of infertility in women. And, with research showing that women struggling with infertility have anxiety and depression rates equal to women with cancer and HIV, it stands to reason that anything we can do to help support our emotional well-being is essential when we're trying to conceive.

One simple step you can take to improve your emotional balance is to make better food choices. Research is beginning to support what any chocolate lover has known for years—food has a profound effect on mood. Let's take a closer look at the intersection of food and brain chemistry to learn how our diet can help us manage our state of mind. Foods, it seems, alter our mood through several different mechanisms: neurotransmitters, endorphins, and satiety.

Neurotransmitters

Neurotransmitters are chemicals that facilitate communication between neurons (nerve cells), allowing information to be sent throughout the brain and body. Neurotransmitters affect physical variables such as heart rate and blood pressure, as well as sleep, the ability to concentrate, and overall mood. Neurotransmitters can be either excitatory or inhibitory. Excitatory neurotransmitters stimulate the brain, while inhibitory neurotransmitters calm the brain. In times of stress and agitation, inhibitory neurotransmitters can become depleted as they strive to "keep the peace."

Three neurotransmitters have been studied extensively in relation to food: dopamine, norepinephrine, and serotonin. Dopamine and norepinephrine are associated with alertness (excitatory), while serotonin is associated with a calming, anti-anxiety effect (inhibitory).

INHIBITORY NEUROTRANSMITTERS: Adequate levels of the inhibitory neurotransmitter serotonin are necessary for a stable mood and to counteract excitatory neurotransmitters in times of stress and stimulation. When brain serotonin levels are stable, our mood is generally balanced. When serotonin fluctuates, we can experience ups and downs in our emotional state.

CARBOHYDRATES cause a short-term increase in serotonin levels and boost mood, which is one reason many people may crave a sugary or potato-chippy snack when they are feeling stressed out or sad. The serotonin/carbohydrate relationship is a double-edged sword, however, as reaching for that sugary snack causes blood sugar to spike, then crash—a setup for an emotional bummer later. Serotonin levels can also be depleted during withdrawal from long-term use of caffeine and stimulants, which explains the temporary depression/blues that accompany getting "off the java." Stress is another condition that depletes serotonin.

EXCITATORY NEUROTRANSMITTERS: Eating protein-rich foods inhibits serotonin production and promotes the production of dopamine and norepinephrine, the two excitatory neurotransmitters. Other factors deplete neurotransmitters, including stress, genetic predisposition, prescription and recreational drugs, and poor diet. The building blocks of neurotransmitters are healthy fats. Studies have shown links between low intakes of omega-3 fatty acids and depression. In addition getting adequate amounts of B vitamins is key for neurotransmitter production.

ENDORPHINS: Endorphins are feel-good neuropeptides that function as neurotransmitters. The brain secrets endorphins as a means of blocking the sensation of pain and producing a feeling of euphoria. Foods that have been shown to increase endorphins include sweet foods, foods rich in fat, and, famously, chocolate. Other healthier sources of endorphins include spicy foods, in particular foods featuring chili peppers. Sex and vigorous exercise are also a great way to stimulate the production of these feel-good chemicals.

SATIETY: Finally, satiety—or how satisfied we are by our meal—can impact mood. After a huge meal, blood is shunted away from the brain to the stomach and digestive organs to aid in digestion. The result? The sluggishness that occurs post-feast. The more fat in a meal (think cheese burger and fries), the longer it takes food to leave the stomach and the longer you may feel drowsy or dopey. On the flip side, meals that are high in processed carbs aren't a great idea, either. These sugars leave the digestive system quickly and hit the bloodstream like a freight train, followed by an inevitable crash and need for another sweet snack.

Mood Management Munchie Tips, or Better Brain Chemistry Through Eating!

1. Meals that have a balanced combination of protein, carbohydrate, and healthy fats are the best choice for an even keel and balanced mood.

2. Make sure your diet has ample sources of omega-3 fatty acids as these are chemical building blocks for neurotransmitters and other important regulatory hormones. Sources of omega-3s include cold-water fatty fish like sardines and wild salmon, walnuts, flax seed, scallops, beans, winter and summer squash, and romaine lettuce. Because women who are trying to conceive are encouraged to limit their consumption of fatty fish, you may also want to consider a high-quality omega-3 supplement.

3. For better energy and clearer thinking before an interview or big presentation, eat a moderately sized meal (400-500 calories) that is rich in lean protein and complemented with whole grains and non-starchy veggies, or try a salad with avocado, walnuts, and lean protein on top.

4. If you're overstimulated at bedtime and need to calm down, try drinking 8 oz of whole milk sweetened with a small amount (½ teaspoon) of honey or agave nectar. Milk is a good source of tryptophan, an amino acid building block for serotonin, and the small amount of sugar will stimulate the quick absorption of tryptophan into the blood and brain.

Once there, tryptophan is converted to serotonin, which itself then regulates melatonin, the sleep-regulating hormone manufactured by the pineal gland, and hey presto! You are swept away to sleepy land. Add a shake of cinnamon if you want to improve blood sugar regulation. If you are avoiding dairy, you can use almond milk to make this bedtime treat, as almonds have a healthy amount of tryptophan as well as the minerals calcium and magnesium which help relax the nervous system.

5. For an endorphin boost, try spicy salsa as a condiment or nibble a piece of chocolate containing at least 70 percent cacao for dessert. Then go have sex—tee hee!

ONE WEEK OF FERTILITY-FRIENDLY EATING

Day	Breakfast	Lunch	Dinner
Mon	Oatmeal with rice milk & raisins, Herbal tea	Baked sweet potato, Steamed broccoli, Orange slices (room temp)	Chicken Stir Fry with Broccoli served over cooked barley, Green peas, Raspberries
Tue	Scrambled eggs with black beans, salsa, and avocado, Herbal tea	Quinoa Vegetable Soup, Rice Crackers	Broiled Salmon, Sweet Potato Fries, Roasted Green Beans, Strawberries w/ whip cream
Wed	Warm amaranth cereal, almond milk, berries, Herbal tea	Turkey breast and avocado slices on whole grain bread, Apple wedges with almond butter	Pasture-raised pork loin, Brown rice or cooked barley, Chocolate-covered walnuts
Thurs	Whole grain bread with cashew butter and a drizzle of agave nectar, Herbal tea	Black bean soup, Avocado slices, Rice cracker	Bison burger served with white bean purée, Roasted Brussels sprouts Warm fruit compote
Fri	Warm apple sauce, Rice cakes with nut butter, Herbal tea	Vegetable Soup, Grapes, Almonds	Pan-fried chicken thighs, Kale sautéed with Sesame and Ginger, Greek yogurt with honey and walnuts
Sat	Oatmeal with rice milk, fruit, and walnuts, Herbal tea	Leftover Chicken in a Pot, Rice Crackers, Plum or nectarine	Vegetable Stew, Brown rice, Cantaloupe slices
Sun	Broiled grapefruit drizzled with agave nectar, "Get Pregnant" granola and whole-milk plain yogurt, Herbal tea	Left-over Quinoa Vegetable Soup Whole grain crackers with salsa or hummus	Baked Tilapia, Roasted Asparagus, Apple and peanut butter

NUTRITIONAL SUPPLEMENTS

In this section we discuss the subject of nutritional supplements. One concern we have about many commercial "cleansing" programs is that they often come with special shakes and may even contain herbs with diuretic and laxative actions. These products are not recommended when you are trying to conceive (and probably even when you're not!).

There are, however, several different nutritional supplements that we do recommend for women who are trying to conceive. Prenatal vitamins are a no-brainer, of course, and are on everyone's pre-conception nutrition checklist. Other supplements, including an omega-3 supplement containing both EPA and DHA essential fatty acids, and a probiotic supplement, promote overall good health, and desirable for their usefulness in limiting chronic inflammation in the body and supporting gut function.

Finally, we discuss several other supplements that are emerging as very useful additions to the field of fertility nutrition, including vitamin D, CoEnzyme Q10, Myo-Inositol, and DHEA.

Note: Proceed with caution. While our "laundry list" of supplements explains the rationale for recommending these supplements for the purposes of supporting fertility, our opinion at Pulling Down the Moon is that you should always consult a nutritionist who is trained in the field of fertility to make sure any supplements you choose are appropriate, given your specific health condition. You should also clear any supplement regimen with your physician.

REQUIRED SUPPLEMENTS

A good quality Prenatal Vitamin (PNV)

Taking a prenatal vitamin (PNV) prior to conception is de rigeur. Even physicians, who are highly skeptical of most supplements, will recommend a PNV to their patient the moment she mentions she is thinking about having a baby. Many women trying to conceive are nutritionally depleted. Some have spent years using oral contraceptives, which deplete the essential B vitamins; others have not paid particular interest to diet and nutrients, such as folic acid and iron, which are absolutely essential for healthy ovulation and pregnancy (adequate folic acid is vital to prevent neural tube defects in the developing embryo). Look for a product that contains minimal fillers and additives, an easily digestible iron (such as ferrous fumarate, ferrous gluconate or ferrous sulfate) and well-absorbed calcium. Some PNVs now contain DHA, one of the omega-3 fatty acids, which supports brain development of the baby in utero.

RECOMMENDED FOR INFLAMMATION, OXIDATIVE STRESS, AND GUT HEALTH

Omega-3 Fatty Acids (with Ample EPA Fatty Acids)

As previously mentioned, many prenatal vitamins these days contain the omega-3 fatty acid DHA to support cognitive development and the central nervous system in the developing baby. EPA is a key component of the body's anti-inflammatory response and has also been shown to be potentially supportive of male fertility and depression. Note: Few prenatal vitamin supplements contain EPA, the omega-3 fatty acid that has been shown to reduce inflammation; you will need to seek them out or supplement in addition to your prenatal.

Look for a pure, high-quality fish oil supplement that provides a daily dose of 1200 mg of the omega-3's EPA and DHA. Look for a breakdown of about 700 mg EPA and 500 mg DHA.

Probiotic Supplement

For all the reasons discussed in Chapter Two and Three of this book, we believe that a probiotic supplement may support fertility and a healthy pregnancy. As we've also seen, maintaining healthy quantities of GI flora in the gut is very important for limiting toxicity. Friendly gut bacteria ensure that metabolic toxins like excess estrogen, which are on their way out of the body, aren't "re-metabolized" by anaerobic organisms in the colon and reabsorbed into the body tissues. Look for a quality-tested probiotic that provides a daily dose of greater than 10 billion organisms.

Whole food "green" beverage

Do you really eat sufficient fruits and vegetables each day? Be honest. As we've discussed, fruit and veg are the best source of many antioxidant nutrient vitamins and minerals, as well as special compounds called flavonoids that are essential to good health. We are not fans of high levels of supplementation with antioxidant vitamins, as studies looking at antioxidant supplementation are not all positive. In fact, several studies have shown increases in cancer risk when antioxidants are supplemented. What is consistent, however, is the link between a diet high in fruits and vegetables and almost every parameter of good health, including fertility. Your Fertility Cleanse eating plan includes lots of fruits and veg, but we all have those days when we just can't seem to get our hands on anything leafy or green. If you are struggling to get adequate servings of veg, a powdered green drink is a nice option, as long as you find one that is made from organic produce and is low in sugar and calories.

"EMERGENT" SUPPLEMENTS: VITAMIN D, COQ10, DHEA, AND MYO-INOSITOL

These next few supplements are ones we choose to use at Pulling Down the Moon because there is preliminary data suggesting they might benefit fertility and little evidence that they can do harm.

Vitamin D

If there were such thing as a "trendy" vitamin, we would have to say that Vitamin D is totally in. In recent years a heated debate has raged over dietary recommendations of this vitamin. Vitamin D, the "sunshine vitamin" manufactured in bare skin exposed to sunlight, is actually a pre-pro-hormone; that means it is a precursor of a precursor of a hormone. Vitamin D deficiency is a chronic issue in modern times due to lower exposure to natural sunlight due to indoor lifestyles and inadequate northerly latitude sunlight (in the United States, that's a line roughly from Boston across the northern part of the country), sunscreens that block UV rays, inadequate vitamin D in diets, and other lifestyle factors, as well as aging and genetic disposition. Vitamin D deficiency is a serious problem because it has been found to be associated with bone fractures, cancer, autoimmune disease, depression, cardiovascular disease, diabetes, and even the flu.

Most important for our purposes, vitamin D may also play an important role in both fertility and pregnancy. Women with higher blood and follicular fluid levels of vitamin D have been shown to be significantly more likely to achieve pregnancy through IVF (Ozkan et al. 2010). Vitamin D deficiency in pregnancy has been associated with increased rates of bacterial vaginosis (which may contribute to miscarriage or preterm birth), and correlates with pre-eclampsia, gestational diabetes, and greater risk of C-section (Hollis et al. 2004).

NOTE: New guidelines from the Food and Nutrition Board recently raised the recommended intake of vitamin D from 200 IU/day to 600 IU/day for adults 19 to 71 years of age, including women who are pregnant or breastfeeding. The safe upper limit is estimated to be 4,000 IUs/day. Your body manufactures roughly 10,000 IUs of vitamin D from 10-15 minutes' exposure of bare skin to sunlight during the middle of the day when all-important UVB sunlight is most plentiful, and overdosing through exposure to sunlight appears not be an issue for humans who evolved with the sun. Supplementation is a very different issue, however. The jury is still out, and you are well advised to take short daily sunbaths and moderately supplement if you are deficient, rather than take megadoses of vitamin D supplements.

The best thing about vitamin D is that through a simple blood test (vitamin D 25-OH) done by your primary care physician, you can find out if you are deficient. If your levels are below 30 ng/ml (per most labs), it is considered a deficiency and you should be supplementing with vitamin D to correct your levels. We generally recommend supplementing vitamin D at 1,000 IU/day (or as directed by your physician), as levels of supplementation below this dosage have not been effective at raising serum vitamin D (Hollis et al 2004).

CoEnzyme Q10 (aka CoQ10)

CoQ10 is a naturally occurring fat-soluble nutrient that is essential for energy production. CoQ10 has potent antioxidant properties and cell membrane stabilizing effects that make it beneficial for egg and sperm quality, specifically sperm motility. CoQ10 works within the mitochondria (the cellular power stations) in the cells and is essential for energy production. Until recently, CoQ10 was not thought to be a nutrient that required supplementation, as all normal tissue manufactures its own CoQ10; however, this production decreases naturally with age and is also lowered by certain drugs, including statins. When CoQ10 levels in the cells are low, energy production may be reduced and oxidative stress increased as a result.

CoQ10 has been shown to improve sperm quality and is now under investigation for potential use with women of advanced reproductive age undergoing ART to improve egg/embryo quality. The oocyte has among the highest concentrations of mitochondria of all body cells and uses immense amounts of energy in the process of maturation and ovulation. Researchers hypothesize that supporting the oocyte with CoQ10 may improve egg quality (Bentov et al. 2010).

The recommended dosage for overall health is 100-300 mg/day, or as directed by a nutritionist. The dosage under investigation in studies looking at egg quality is higher: 600 mg/day. CoQ10 appears to be a safe supplement: Studies have used supplementation of CoQ10 up to levels of 3,000 mg per day without adverse side effects. At present, the only risk to taking CoQ is the cost, as this supplement can be pricy, and no data currently exists on its usage in high doses during pregnancy.

Dehydroepiandrosterone (DHEA)

DHEA (short for dehydroepiandrosterone) is not to be confused with the omega-3 fatty acid DHA, although they sound alike. DHA is a fatty acid, whereas DHEA is precursor to hormones manufactured in the adrenal glands and one of the most abundant circulating hormones in the human body.

DHEA has recently garnered a lot of attention in the world of fertility for helping women with Decreased Ovarian Reserve (DOR) and Premature Ovarian Failure (POF), as it is a precursor to hormones such as testosterone and estrogens and may help increase follicular stimulation. It is also known to sharply decline with age. DHEA has been shown in some small studies to improve IVF outcomes in women that are poor responders to IVF (Wiser et al., 2010) Some research also points to DHEA as possibly reducing aneuploidy (chromosomal abnormalities) in embryos, and thereby decreasing miscarriage rates (Gleicher et al., 2010).

Most studies have been carried out using DHEA supplementation of 25-75 mg/day. A few things should be noted about utilizing DHEA when trying to conceive. First, it should not be taken in high doses for a long period as it may cause undesirable fluctuations in hormone levels and may also cause liver damage. Also, before beginning DHEA, it is advisable to get DHEA-S levels tested to make sure they are within range before supplementation. We also strongly encourage you to notify your Reproductive Endocrinologist before supplementing with DHEA. Unlike the omega-3 fat DHA, DHEA is NOT to be used if pregnant and should be discontinued as soon as a positive pregnancy test is achieved. DHEA should also not be used if you have PCOS, as this hormone may make this condition worse. DHEA is available over the counter at low cost.

Myo-Inositol

Myo-inositol is a B vitamin that has been utilized as an insulin sensitizer in women with Polycystic Ovarian Syndrome (POS). Myo-inositol can be synthesized by the body from other nutrients, but when deficient it can impact the body's sensitivity to insulin. Research shows that when myo-inositol is taken daily, it can help to restore ovulation and menstruation in some women. Supplementation with myo-inositol has been clinically shown to lower levels of circulating insulin and testosterone, promote ovulation, improve egg quality, improve hirsutism and acne, and lower the risk of ovarian hyperstimulation syndrome (OHSS) during an IVF cycle. Some research has found it to be as clinically effective as Metformin in restoring ovulation (Papeleo et al., 2009).

Recommended dosage for supplementation is 4 g per day. Another closely related and popular supplement for PCOS is D-Chiro Inositol (DCI). There are actually nine different forms of inositol (part of B-complex vitamins), with DCI and myo-inositol being the two most researched in conjunction with insulin sensitivity. As we mentioned previously, most of the research on fertility/PCOS has used the myo- form of inositol. For this reason, and because DCI can be a bit more pricy, we use myo-inositol at Pulling Down the Moon.

BASELINE NUTRITION WORKSHEET

	Day 1	Day 2	Day 3	Day 4	Day 5	Day 6	Day 7
Date							
Wake Up:							
Morning Meal:							
Time:							
Snack:							
Time:							
Evening Meal:							
Time:							
Water (Ounces):							
Other:							
Activity/ Exercise:							
What Kind:							
How Long:							
Sleep Time:							

CHAPTER 9

The Cleansing Power of Water

Water is a very powerful symbol for the purposes of the Fertility Cleanse Lifestyle. It is necessary for the existence of life—it flows effortlessly, washes away the dirt, quenches our thirst, encompasses the majority of our planet, and can be found in plenty throughout our own bodies. Water can be used to cool us when we are hot and heat us when we are cold. While most of us associate bathing with personal hygiene, early records show that the bath may have originally been used for ritualistic or religious purposes to purify the spirit. In many cultures water was—and still is—a symbol for washing away sin or imperfection. Total submersion in water has been seen as a mini-death, then rebirth or rejuvenation. In the Christian tradition, for example, it is used as a symbol in baptismal rites of being born into the family of God.

In the early stages of development, amniotic fluid is primarily made of water supplied by the mother. A fetus breathes amniotic fluid in the womb, which helps with lung development and is later excreted as urine. It also surrounds and protects the developing fetus from crushing blows.

Throughout history, water has also been seen as magical, its source coming from some supreme deity. Ask Native Americans in the bone-dry Southwest, whose most significant dances are directed at rain gods, or the Biblical Moses, who parted the Red Sea, or the Hindus who submerge themselves in the Ganges for purification. Noah built his ark to avoid the Great Flood and the wrath of God. The water, in this case, is perhaps seen as a divine punishment from which Noah survives because of his moral worthiness. The flood washed away the sins of the world so that we could start anew.

In yoga, the yogi believes there is nothing standing between us and the Creator, except our own forgetfulness. We forget that the Creator is within us. We think of this Source as being "somewhere out there" rather than "right here." We begin to feel separated from this Source and unworthy. We see the Source as pure and clean and ourselves as dirty or toxic. For these reasons, the Fertility Cleanse Lifestyle includes three cleansing water practices: The first is drinking water, the second is using water to cleanse our sinus passages, and the third includes ritual bathing.

Drinking Water

It is well known that more than 60 percent of our body weight is compromised of water. We lose water every day through urination, sweat, breathing, and regular cellular activity. When we do not replenish this natural water loss, the body's metabolism can slow down and the process of toxin removal, healing, removal of old cells, and replacement with new tissues can become compromised. Drinking water is an important part of the cleansing process and helps support the detoxification process in the liver.

In addition to supporting your organs of detoxification, drinking extra water during this time offers other benefits. Your skin may become less dry, you may be less prone to acne, your bowel movements might become more regular, and your nose and throat membrane may feel moist or more thoroughly lubricated. For those of you currently taking fertility medications, a little extra H2O during this time can help decrease that bloated feeling you maybe experiencing with the drugs.

Water is essential in supporting proper functioning in the body. For instance, water helps with the transportation of hormones, nutrients, oxygen, and antibodies throughout the bloodstream and lymphatic system. Water is also present during the digestion process, which helps with the breakdown and absorption of solid foods. Water can also benefit our physical appearance by helping hydrate cells, making the skin look plumper and less saggy.

The amount of water you need daily can vary widely depending on your body size, how much you exercise, where you live, or your health condition. As a general rule of thumb, you should drink enough water so that your urine is pale yellow rather than dark. The color of your urine is a good indicator as to whether or not you are properly hydrated. During your Fertility Cleanse program, we suggest you increase your intake of room temp or warm water, but don't overdo it. When your kidneys are unable to excrete the excess water, the electrolyte (mineral) content of the blood is diluted, resulting in low sodium levels in the blood and faulty cellular metabolism, a condition called hyponatremia. This condition causes the cells in your body to swell which can result in a myriad of problems from mild fatigue to severe muscle weakness, decreased consciousness or even coma. First aid for this condition can include mixing 1/8 teaspoonful of sea salt in a glass of water to keep cells balanced.

During your fertility cleanse, water should be consumed at meal time in place of sugary fruit juices or soda pop which is void of nutritional value. Water should also be consumed between meals, and especially before and after exercising. Sparkling water with a twist of lemon in a fancy glass makes a nice substitute for alcoholic beverages at social gatherings.

With so many different types of water available on the market today, it is sometimes difficult knowing which one to buy. Our position is that any mineral or spring water is fine for drinking, but you should consider staying away from large amounts of bottled water. Plastic bottles contain significant quantities of BPA, a known toxin that can often leach from the bottle into the water, and into you. It is best to get yourself a water filter for your kitchen tap or a water pitcher with a built-in filter and simply and inexpensively refill a reusable steel drinking bottle to carry with you (they are now widely available).

Distilled water is another "no-no." Water made through the distillation process has been purified through evaporation and, in the process, has been stripped of most naturally occurring minerals. Magnesium, calcium, iron, and other minerals found in water are important for your fertility and the future health of your baby, so refrain from purchasing water of the distilled variety.

Our goal for the Fertility Cleansing Lifestyle is to support liver function and excretion of toxins. Your liver functions as a filter, so optimal blood volume will help this organ do its job more efficiently. If you do not regularly flush metabolic waste out of your body, you may feel a bit sick, sluggish, or feel headache pain (see box on Ama Cleanse). While the amount of water suggested above will send you to the toilet frequently for elimination, over time as your body gets used to this additional fluid intake, you will find your stops to the restroom less frequent. Remember, this exercise calls for pure drinking water. Drinking soda, coffee, or lemonade is not the same. If you feel sick of plain water, you may squeeze in some fresh lemon, cucumber, or grind up fresh mint or ginger for a hot tea. Thoroughly wash anything you add to your hot water, and remember that ingredients need to be pure and caffeine free. These simple teas can be counted toward your 10-12 cups of daily water intake. High-quality herbal teas are okay as long as the herbs are not meant for medicinal purposes.

Ama Cleanse

Sometimes our bodies are not able to digest or absorb all food matter, particularly when the food contains preservatives, additives, chemicals, or is grown in an environment using herbicides, pesticides, growth hormones, or antibiotics. According to the traditional Indian medical science of Ayurveda, frozen foods, processed foods, alcohol, caffeine, nicotine, fried foods, candy, and white sugared foods are all food items that do not always get thoroughly digested, absorbed, or eliminated by the body. Other foods we eat may not be suited to our constitution, such as gluten for those with celiac disease.

Yogis believe that when the body is unable to thoroughly process these foods, a residue is left behind that becomes the building block for imbalance in the digestive system. This residue is called ama, and it can be likened to a mass of gunk that starts to line the stomach, digestive tract, or even arteries, causing a clog in the flow of energy. If not flushed away, ama can create a toxic buildup and becomes a fertile breeding ground for inflammation, disease, infection, or illness to take root and flourish.

In both Ayurveda and Traditional Chinese Medicine (TCM), it is believed that drinking iced water or ice-cold beverages douses the digestive fire and causes ama to be generated. For the purposes of your new cleanse lifestyle, it is recommended that only room temperature or hot water be consumed.

For a simple Ama cleanse, drink 8 cups of hot water (as hot as you can stand it) with a squeeze of fresh lemon daily for seven days.

Nasal Cleansing/Neti Pot

The jala neti, or nasal wash, is an old yogic technique used to irrigate the nasal passages and sinuses and rid them of extra mucus, allergens, and germs. Nasal washing has proven to be effective in the treatment of chronic sinonasal symptoms. While the technique is very old, it has enjoyed a resurgence in popularity, as research has shown daily saline nasal irrigation decreases sinus symptoms and medication use in patients with frequent sinusitis and improves quality of life (Rabago D. Et al., 2006).

Many doctors today recommend their patients use a saline nasal spray for the moistening and cleansing of the nasal passages. They often refer patients to their local drugstore or pharmacy for purchase of these products. It is our belief that over-the-counter products are unnecessary, costly, and less effective than the use of a good, old-fashioned neti pot, now easily available online or at your local wellness store. A neti pot is typically made of glass, metal, ceramic, or heavy plastic. It looks like a small, squatty watering can with a long, narrow spout that fit inside the nostril.

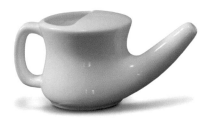

The basic premise of nasal irrigation using a neti pot is for saline water to travel in one nostril and out the other (with the more adept practitioner, the water can exit out of the mouth). Each of us has probably experienced the discomfort of accidentally snorting water from the pool or bathtub, which leaves our noses in a burning or painful stupor and causes our eyes to water uncontrollably. Thankfully, the nasal wash feels nothing like this. While the process may sound intimidating, within a few short days you can become a neti pot pro and wow all your friends at your next dinner party with your amazing water breathing feat.

Over time, you will find your nasal wash becomes a regular part of your day and without it, your snout will just not feel quite right. We recommend you use your neti pot every single day as part of your bathing or shower ritual.

Simple Directions for your Daily Nasal Cleanse

Many folks go to extravagant lengths to buy special salts, solutions, or drops for their neti pot. We prefer to keep it pure and simple, using the following technique:

STEP 1:

While in the shower, fill your neti pot with warm water from your shower head or tap.

STEP 2:

Add uniodized salt, as directed by the manufacturer of your neti pot. Uniodized salt is basically pure salt without the addition of iodine. It can be easily found in your grocery store and is usually priced under a dollar for a large tub. Typically speaking, the perfect water to salt ratio is ¾-teaspoon of salt to 16 ounces of water. Since neti pots vary in size, we recommend you use the salt/water ratio as recommended by the manufacturer of your neti pot, or get a gallon of distilled water and add salt, using the ratio prescribed above. You will find that over time, once you get a feel for your neti pot, you will simply be able to fill your pot with tap water, and estimate your salt usage with your fingers.

Tami's Neti Story

Before I left my job in advertising I was suffering from chronic sinus infections. I don't know whether I was so stressed that my immune system was compromised at the time, or whether I was never really able to get rid of one infection which, ultimately, led to the next. What I do know is that I couldn't breathe, I had constant sinus pain, and I felt absolutely miserable; it was like a bad cold that never went away.

I had made several trips to the doctor's office and went through several rounds of antibiotics and even steroids to help reduce the swelling in the sinus cavities. I would get better for a short amount of time and then the infection would reoccur. In desperation, I went to an Ear, Nose and Throat specialist, who did a CT scan of my sinuses. He called me in for a consultation and said that every single one of my sinuses had scar tissue and damage, which meant that I would need surgery if I was ever going to feel better.

Before scheduling the surgery he suggested I go on a 30-day course of antibiotics. During this time, I decided to try the ancient yoga tradition of sinus washing.

I bought a neti pot, some uniodized salt, and set to work with my nose bidet in a last-ditch effort to save myself from surgery. I used the neti pot every single day. Miraculously, I started feeling better. The long-term course of antibiotics combined with the neti pot helped me avoid surgery. In the 10 years since that time, I have had only one sinus infection. In fact, the daily use of my neti pot has lessened the symptoms of seasonal allergies and makes recovery time from the common cold and other illnesses quite speedy.

There have been times when it has been nearly impossible to use the neti. During bad colds or times when nasal passages are inflamed, it is very challenging to get water through them. I stick with it, though. Just getting water into the nose can be a very soothing experience when you aren't feeling your best. I have been using the neti pot daily for over a decade now and am convinced it has been an inexpensive, pure, and easy way for me to avoid surgery, recover more quickly from illness, and keep me feeling healthy. It is one of the best investments you can make in your holistic health.

The Cleansing Bath

Bathing rituals are another important part of the Cleanse Lifestyle. They represent a purification and rebirthing process that allows us to clean ourselves from the outside in. This occurs first by cleansing the physical body of its impurities, then by clearing the mental body of its erroneous thoughts, and finally by purifying our spiritual body so that we may remember our unity with the Source (Awareness).

It is easy to understand how a cleansing bath might benefit the physical body: It gets rid of germs, opens our pores, soothes our muscles, and induces the Relaxation Response. It's more difficult to understand how a simple bath might purify erroneous thoughts or help bring us spiritual peace. Remember, the value of a ritual is that it symbolically helps bring about a different state of consciousness. First, the water works on a physical level by encouraging the body to say, "Ooh, this feels good. I'm very relaxed." Once the body is relaxed, and we tell our mind we are doing a ritual, we take on a different, more aware state of consciousness. It is during this state of heightened Awareness that we allow ourselves to open up to the healing process of the ritual. By bringing intention and attention into our bath, we can more easily surrender to the feeling inside the water. We let our muscles go, allow the water to support us, and permit our thoughts to melt away—just like the fetus floating effortlessly in the amniotic fluid of the womb.

It is virtually impossible to do justice in the space available here to all the different types of water rituals that exist in the world. They are many, and may include immersion, splashing, sprinkling, showering, or dousing, depending on the religion, culture, or history behind the bath. We encourage you to continue your exploration of spiritual bathing; you may find a ritual that is particularly meaningful to you. To support your fertility, keep in mind that extreme hot or extreme cold water is not recommended, nor is the use of very exotic herbs, essences, flowers, or other plant material that might be contraindicated for fertility or good vaginal health.

To get you started, we have included two different "recipes" for a cleansing bath in this book that are fertility friendly. One is a safe yet simple cleansing bath and the other is a vaginal steam bath.

Cleansing baths are recommended before you start a new medical cycle or if you did not have success with an old one. In fact, it could also be used as the "opening ceremony" for your Cleanse Lifestyle as outlined in this book. The bath can also be used to help clear away a negative experience or memory you hold within. It is also recommended after miscarriage, during or right after your menses, or while taking a break from medical treatment. If you are having difficulty with your partner, if you are not seeing eye to eye, or if you are looking for a way to put closure to a challenging event, consider bathing together. Cleansing baths are not encouraged post-ovulation if you think you could be pregnant.

An important factor in spiritual bathing is the ambience of the room where you are bathing. Part of the ritual is allowing the water to soothe you, so it is important that you do your bath at a time when you are assured it will be peaceful and without interruption.

Setting the Stage for your Cleansing Bath

We recommend you do the bathing ritual at night, just before bedtime, to help optimize relaxation and allow the ritual to settle into deeper awareness while you sleep.

- Fill the tub with water. Allow the water to be hot enough so that you will still be comfortable in the tub after sitting for 20-30 minutes, but not so hot that getting into the tub water feels uncomfortably hot. As the tub fills, add the following to your cleansing bath:
- 1 pound of Epsom salts or sea salt
- 1 box of baking soda
- Dim the lights and let the bathroom glow with soft candlelight. Have a robe or towel close by to avoid getting chilled when you finish this ritual. Soft, relaxing music is permissible. After entering the water, and once completely submerged, recite the following invocation:

    I now begin a physical, mental, and spiritual cleanse. Give me strength to see through this process the Self inside me that needs no cleansing—to awaken to the fact that I am already happy, healthy, and whole in this very moment. Grant that through this process my body also awakens to greater health and well-being by my own self-discipline, pure-hearted intention, and respect for this physical form I have been given.

- Sit in the tub for 20-30 minutes. Be careful when you stand up. Then shower or rinse your body thoroughly.

Note: This is a highly concentrated solution of salt and soda. While you can repeat the bath frequently, you should not do the cleansing solution of sea salt and baking soda more than once a month.

CHAPTER 10

The Cleansing Power of Yoga

In Chapter Four we delved deeply into the ways that yoga can promote radiant health, support fertility and protect the body from the ravages of stress and the environment. But talking about yoga and doing yoga are not the same thing. Now it is time to practice. If you read our previous book, *Fully Fertile*, you will be familiar with the posture sequences presented in this section. With this new understanding of the way yoga works to detoxify body and mind, you can practice these poses as part of your cleanse program.

For best results, we recommend that you practice yoga a minimum of 3 times per week for approximately 30-45 minutes at a time. Feel free to combine any of the yoga exercises, but as a general rule each practice should start with Moon Salutes and end with Svasana (Resting Pose).

It is our experience that most women are comfortable with this practice throughout their ART cycles and into pregnancy. As always, however, discuss your exercise program with your doctor to ensure it is appropriate for you.

Kriya (Cleansing) Exercises

Kriya are cleansing exercises that help to dislodge toxicity and open important energy channels. These particular kriya are fertility-specific and stimulate the musculature and fascia of the low back, hips, and the feet, opening the apana energy channel. Hips and feet are linked to the downward flow of energy that helps to ground us and make us feel emotionally secure. These exercises can be done daily.

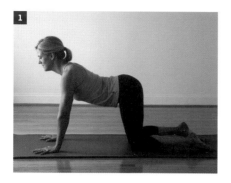

CHAKRA VRKSASANA

Chakra Vrksasana is a wonderful warm-up for the low back, hips, and breath. This three-part kriya exercise is done in two phases:

1. Begin in Table Pose, on your hands and knees
2. Take a deep inhale and then exhale, round your back like an angry cat and sit your seat back on to your heels (Child Pose).
3. With your next inhale, return to Table Pose.

Repeat 4 times, using your breath to set the pace of the movement.

Try to take your time moving between Table Pose and Child Pose, feeling the spine as it rounds and the muscles of the back becoming warm. Feel how the breath and the movement become synchronized.

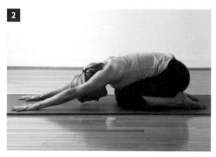

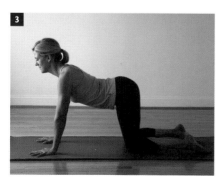

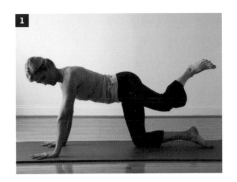

HIP CIRCLES

1. From Table Pose, lift the right leg with knee bent 90 degrees and make full circles in the hip joint. Do this with the intention of "clearing out cobwebs" in the hip sockets. Rest in Child Pose.
2. Bring your awareness to the sole of the right foot. Perhaps it is more "alive" than before.
3. Now move the left side. Bring your awareness to the sole of the left foot. Perhaps it is more "alive" than before.

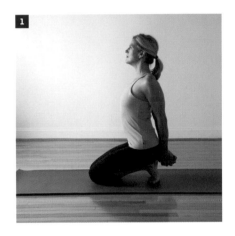

STRETCHING THE SOLE

1. Stand on your knees, curl toes under and sit your seat back gently on to the heels. If the soles of your feet or your toes are very tight, this may be quite uncomfortable. Never force, go gently. The soles of the feet are important conduits for apana energy, the energy that supports fertility.
2. Next, move back into Table and gently tap the tops of the feet on the floor, massaging and encouraging blood and energy flow into tight toes and ankles.

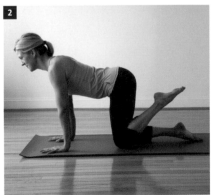

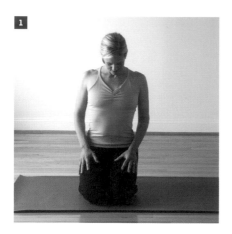

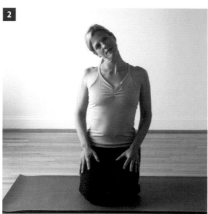

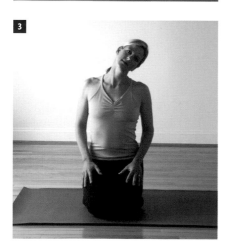

NECK ROLLS

1. Gently drop your head, chin to chest.
2. Now make a soft arc to the right, drawing the right ear towards the right shoulder. Linger in any part of the range of motion that feels tight or tense.
3. Gently roll to the other side.

Repeat.

ASANA PRACTICES

Once you have completed these Kriya (Cleansing) Exercises, it is time to "build" your yoga asana practice, which should consist of:

- PDtM Moon Salutes (2–4 rounds)
- One of the therapeutic sessions—Hip/Heart Opening or Digestion/Hormonal Balance

After this you will enter the last section of Yoga for Fertility practice, the relaxation phase. This is also known as the Final Resting Pose or Svasana (5–10 minutes).

Moon Salutes

The PDtM practice begins with 2–4 rounds PDtM's Moon Salutes. This series of postures, which links breath and movement, effects a gentle warming in the body as well as helps to transition the mind into a more meditative state. The linking of breath and movement is called vinyasa and as you become more adept with your yoga practice you may actually feel your breath beginning to lead your body from pose to pose. As opposed to the more commonly known and more vigorous Surya Namaskar (Sun Salutation), this moon salute uses squats, folds, and lunges to stimulate blood flow into the pelvis and legs, to calm the mind and to strengthen apana vayu.

Do 2–4 rounds of Moon Salutes (one round = once through on each side). Focus on the ujayii breath and the flow of postures. From your final Tadasana (Mountain) Pose go directly into the therapeutic session of your choice.

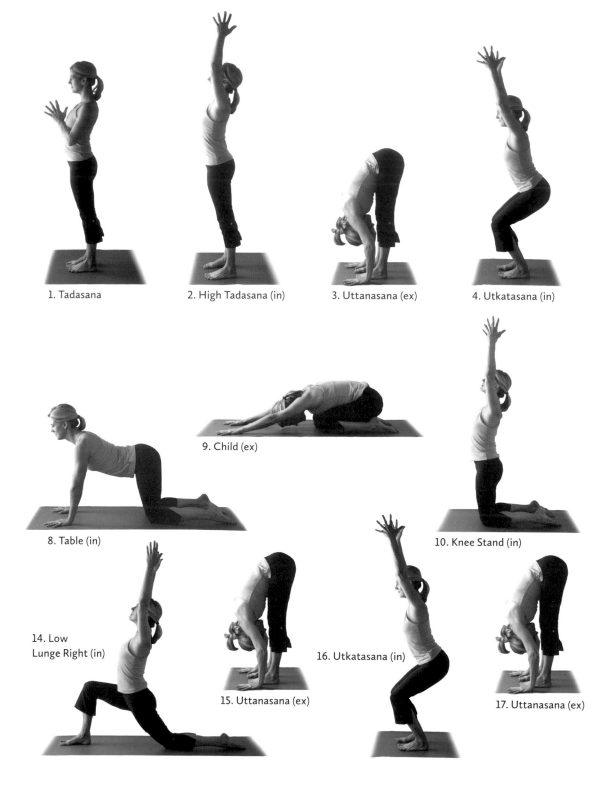

1. Tadasana

2. High Tadasana (in)

3. Uttanasana (ex)

4. Utkatasana (in)

9. Child (ex)

8. Table (in)

10. Knee Stand (in)

14. Low Lunge Right (in)

15. Uttanasana (ex)

16. Utkatasana (in)

17. Uttanasana (ex)

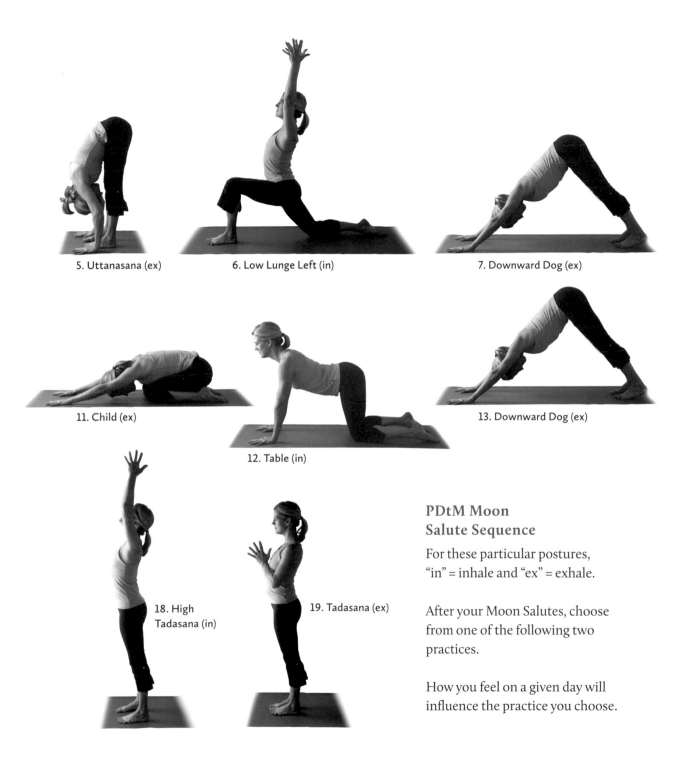

5. Uttanasana (ex)

6. Low Lunge Left (in)

7. Downward Dog (ex)

11. Child (ex)

12. Table (in)

13. Downward Dog (ex)

18. High
Tadasana (in)

19. Tadasana (ex)

PDtM Moon Salute Sequence

For these particular postures, "in" = inhale and "ex" = exhale.

After your Moon Salutes, choose from one of the following two practices.

How you feel on a given day will influence the practice you choose.

Asana Practice 1: Hips and Heart Opening
Apana/Prana Practice

The first practice to open hips and heart includes standing postures to ground the energy in the legs and feet and improve the flow of apana energy in the body. This practice also uses shoulder stretches and supported backbends to release anxiety.

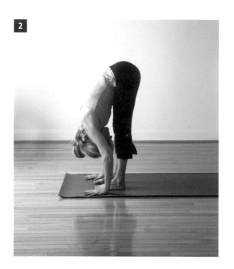

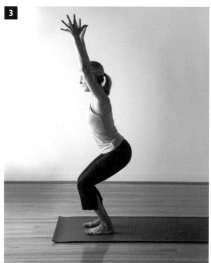

UTTANASANA/UTKATASANA VINYASA

1. Stand with your feet hip-distance apart at the top of your mat, hands on hips.
2. Inhale, then with your exhale, hinge forward into Forward Fold. Knees will be bent or straight, depending on your hamstring flexibility.
3. With your next inhale, bend your knees and sit your seat into Chair Pose. Hold for 3 breaths.

Repeat 2 more times.

This vinyasa helps to build a gentle heat (tapas) in the body as well as strengthen the apana vayu. The forward fold releases tension in the lower back and stimulates the second chakra, or fertility chakra.

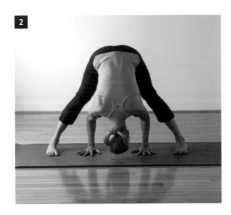

PRASARITA PADOTTANASANA WITH SQUATS

1. Stand with your feet spread wide on your mat, feet parallel.
2. Inhale, then fold forward into Prasarita Padottanasana. Hold here and breathe for several breaths.
3. Now walk your hands forward about 2 feet and gently press your weight back in space.
4. With an inhale, take a squat in Prasarita Padottanasana.

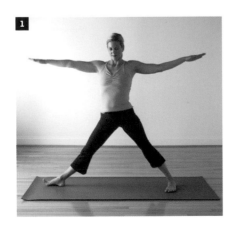

The squat may be a small movement, depending on hip flexibility, and it may feel like you're just plain stuck. Don't judge, just observe the sensation as it arises.

Focus on the breath as you repeat sequence 2–3 times.

This vinyasa stretches hamstrings, groin muscles, and deep hip flexors. Notice how your hips "hum" when you're finished with this one.

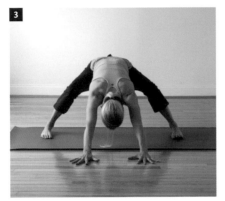

DYNAMIC VIRABHADRASANA II

1. From the previous pose, turn your right toes out 90 degrees, and angle your left toes towards the right. Check your alignment. If you drew a line from the right heel to the left foot it would bisect the left arch. Extend arms out in opposite directions, shoulder height.

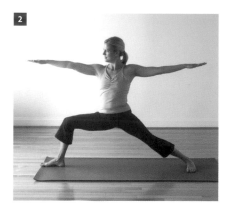

2. Take an inhale, and with your next exhale, bend your right knee 90 degrees.

Repeat 4 times on the right side, inhaling the right leg straight, exhaling right knee bent. Now do the other side.

Virabhadrasana II translates as Warrior Pose. This is a fabulous fertility pose. In addition to stimulating apana, it also helps to strengthen and stretch the muscles of our legs. This pose also challenges us to find the subtle balance between hard work and effortlessness.

TRIKONASANA

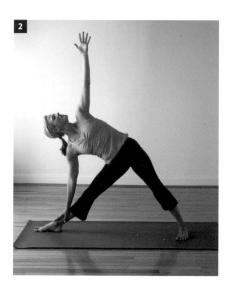

1. From Virabhadrasana II, straighten your right leg and narrow your stance a bit. Again, turn your right toes out 90 degrees, and angle your left toes towards the right.
2. Take an inhale and with your exhale, place the right hand down on your shin, extending the left hand skyward. Take 5–10 breaths.

Repeat on the other side.

Trikonasana stretches hips, groin, and low back. In addition, the pose is a wonderful heart opener and reduces chronic tension in the upper back.

NUMBER FOUR/SUPTA HASTA PADANGUSTHASANA

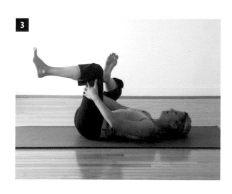

This pose is called Number Four Pose because the leg configuration resembles the number "4." To do the pose:
1. Lay on your back with your knees bent, feet on the floor, hip-distance apart.
2. Cross your right ankle on to your left knee.
3. Now lift your left foot (bottom leg) off the floor and draw the left thigh towards the body.

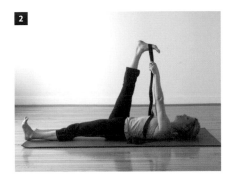

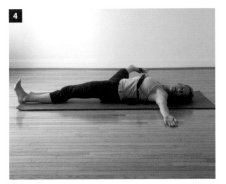

You can interlace your fingers behind the left thigh to help encourage the stretch. You should not feel this in the knee of the crossed leg. If you do, place the bottom foot back on the ground and enjoy the stretch here. Hold for 10–20 deep breaths.

Now move into Supta Hasta Padangusthasana:

1. Stretch your left leg along the floor and put your yoga strap around the sole of the right foot. Extend the foot to the ceiling.
2. Gently stretch the leg as straight as possible without straining, and flex the right foot.
3. Hold 5–10 breaths.
4. Now take both ends of the strap into the right hand and lower the right leg out to the side until you feel a good stretch in the right inner thigh. Keep left hip/buttocks grounded.
5. Hold for 5–10 breaths.
6. Bring leg back up and hug it into your chest.

Repeat series beginning with the Number Four Pose on the left side.

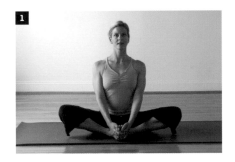

BADDHA KONASANA

1. Sit up straight with the soles of your feet touching, knees apart (you can sit on a folded blanket if it is difficult to sit on the floor with a straight spine).
2. Take hold of the feet with your hands. Inhale, sit up straight and tall, and exhale, folding forward. Keep your spine as straight as possible as you hinge from the hips. Take 5–10 breaths here.

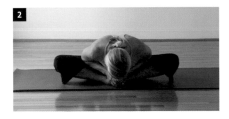

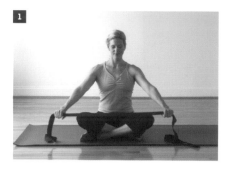

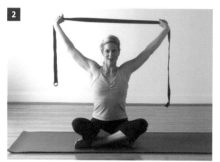

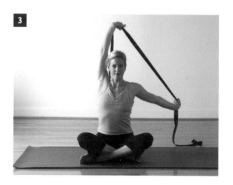

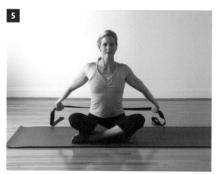

SHOULDER SERIES WITH STRAP

1. Sit in a comfortable seated position and take your yoga strap in both hands, hands about shoulders' width apart.
2. With an inhale, stretch the strap up over your head. Take 5–10 breaths as you stretch your arms gently up and back.
3. Drop the right arm down and bring the left arm up, taking 5–10 breaths. Return arms over head. Now let's try the other side. Take the right arm down and bring the left arm up taking 5-10 breaths.
4. Lower arms to the front as in picture 1.

Now try the "Up-and-Over" Shoulder Stretch:

5. With the same shoulder-width grip on the strap, inhale the arms up and overhead and then exhale the strap down behind your back.
7. Inhale and take the strap overhead, returning to the starting point, as in photo 2.

The goal of the up-and-over is to keep the arms straight during the entire range of movement. If you cannot take the strap up and over with straight arms, take a wider grip on the strap. Go slow, take your time at the "sticky" parts and enjoy the sensation as you open tight chest muscles and rediscover lost shoulder mobility.

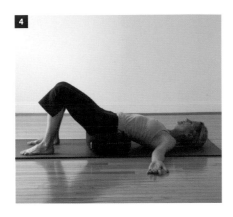

SUPPORTED SETU BANDHASANA

1. Lie on your back with your knees bent, feet flat on the floor, hip-distance apart.
2. Lift your hips and slide a bolster or 2 rolled blankets under the small of your back and lower hips down. The bolster should support the lower back and there should be no discomfort in the sacral area.
3. Take arms out to the sides, palms facing up.
4. Breathe and fully surrender to gravity and allow the bolster to support and nurture your lower back. Deeply release in the pelvis and buttocks. Hold here up to 5 minutes.

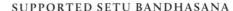

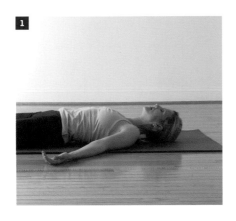

RELAXATION, OR SVASANA

Svasana is the most important pose of our yoga practice. In Svasana all the physical, energetic, and emotional work of practice is processed and our bodies have time to rest and restore. It is a time of profound "not-doing" as well as an opportunity to surrender to something greater than ourselves.

1. Lie on your back, legs and arms straight, palms facing up. If the lower back feels uncomfortable in this position, place a bolster under your knees.
2. Starting at your feet, scan your body for any residual tension. If you find any places that are restless or tense, breathe into them and allow them to relax with your exhale.
3. Let go of the effort of being in the physical body. Allow your body to become very heavy.
4. Let go of the effort of breathing. Release the ujayii breath and let the breath breathe you.
5. Let go of effort of thought. Choose not to attach to the thoughts that wander through your head.
6. Now let everything go—body, mind and spirit— surrendering to the present moment.

Asana Practice 2: Hormonal Regulation/Digestion Improvement
Samana Practice

The goal of this practice is to balance the endocrine system, improve digestion and the assimilation of nutrients (samana vayu) as well as speed up the elimination of toxins. The gentle twists in this practice are safe for the fertility process and will help to release tension in the abdomen, improve blood flow to the abdominal region and stimulate digestion.

Shoulder Stand and Supported Fish stimulate the thyroid gland by first compressing (Shoulder Stand), then stretching (Supported Fish) the throat area. The thyroid gland is essential for good hormonal function and strong metabolism. Practicing Shoulder Stand in this way is also quite calming, and it stimulates our body's "rest and digest" hormone system. This is also known as the autonomic hormone system.

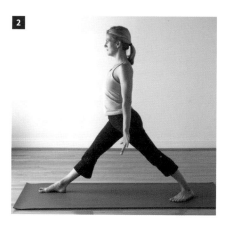

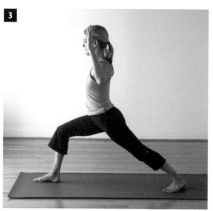

DYNAMIC VIRABHADRASANA I

Also known as Warrior I, this standing pose creates strength and flexibility in the hips, shoulders, and upper back. As you practice the dynamic vinyasa, you may feel heat building in your body.

1. Stand, feet together, at the front of your mat. Take a big step backward with your left foot, about 3½ feet.
2. Keep your right toes facing forward, angle left toes slightly left, about 45 degrees. Hands hang down at your sides. Try to square your hips forward.
3. With an inhale, bend the right knee as close to 90 degrees as possible. At the same time, raise your arms to a "double cactus" position, elbows bent and palms facing forward.
4. Exhale and straighten the right leg, lowering arms. Repeat this 5 times and on the last repetition, hold bent leg position and take 10 breaths.

Repeat on the left.

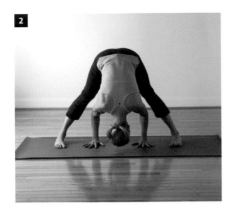

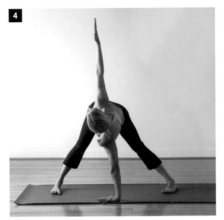

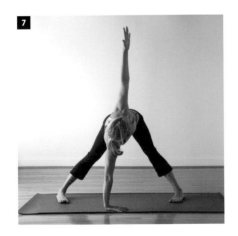

PRASARITA PADOTTANASANA WITH TWIST
Also known as Wide Leg Forward Bend, this pose stretches the groin and hamstrings. When we add the twist element, we make the spine more supple as well as stimulate the abdominal organs.

1. Stand with feet spread wide on your mat, feet parallel.
2. Inhale, then fold forward into Wide Leg Forward Bend. Hold here and take several breaths.
3. Place your left hand on the floor under your nose, with your fingers facing to the right. You can place your hand on a block if you have difficulty keeping your knees straight.
4. With an inhale, stretch your right hand up to the sky, gently twisting in the upper back. As you breathe here, try and stack the right shoulder directly above the left.
5. Press down into both feet, reach back through your tailbone and forward through the crown of your head. Find the current of energy that runs from the left hand up through the right fingertips.
6. Take 5–10 breaths. Release to center with an exhale. Rest a moment and enjoy the sensation.
7. Now place the right hand on the floor (or on a block) under your nose and reach skyward with the left. Again, locate all the currents of energy flowing here, downward through the soles of the feet, along the spine from the tailbone to head and through the heart from palm to palm.
8. Take 5–10 breaths here and then release again to center.

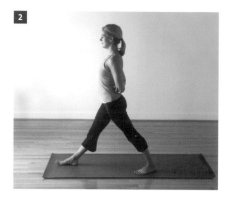

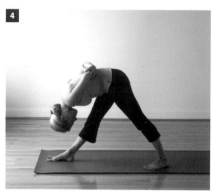

PARSVOTTANASANA

You may find you struggle with balance in this pose, which is also called Pyramid Pose. This standing asana stretches hips, hamstrings, and low back. In addition, the forward fold nourishes and stimulates the lower abdomen and belly.

1. Stand at the front of your mat, feet together. Take a step backward with your left foot, about 2½ feet.
2. Keep your right toes facing forward, turn the left toes out about 45 degrees to the left. Square hips forward.
3. Reach your arms out to the sides with an inhale and with your exhale, grab opposite elbows behind your back.
4. Inhale and then exhale, allowing your torso to fold forward into Parsvottanasana. Keep squaring your hips forward. Breathe here for 5–10 breaths.
5. With an inhale, come up with a straight spine.

Repeat other side.

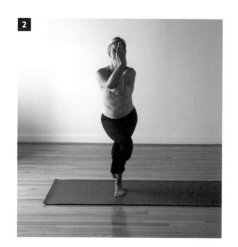

GARUDASANA (EAGLE POSE)

Eagle pushes blood from the extremities into the abdomen, nourishing organs of digestion and reproduction. It detoxifies by compressing lymph nodes in the armpits and groin.

1. From standing, bend your left knee slightly and shift weight into the left leg and lift the right leg up, wrapping the right thigh around the left, hooking the right foot behind the left ankle.
2. Now bend your elbows and lift them to shoulder level. Cross the left elbow over the right and hook the right wrist and palm over the left. Hold for 10 breaths.

Repeat other side.

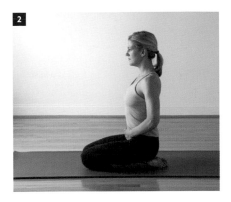

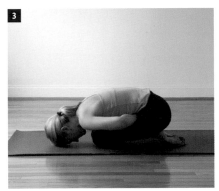

VADHRASANA WITH ABDOMINAL MASSAGE

Omit this pose if you are taking ovarian stimulation drugs, are post-ovulation, post-retrieval, or if there is any chance that you may be pregnant.

1. Come into a kneeling position, tops of the feet on the floor beneath your seat. If you experience discomfort in your knees or the tops of the feet you may place a blanket under your seat.
2. Make fists with your hands and place them in the crease between your thigh and torso.
3. Inhale and then exhale your torso forward over your fists.
4. Gently move the fists around in circles, kneading the lower abdomen.
5. Inhale, come back up, and move the fists higher so the knuckles meet in front of the navel.
6. Inhale and with an exhale fold forward again, this time using the compressed fists to gently massage the middle of the belly.
7. Inhale, come back up, and shift the fists higher on the belly so that they rest on the fleshy part of the belly just below the ribcage.
8. With your next exhale, fold forward again, massaging the upper abdomen just below the diaphragm muscle.
9. Inhale back to seated and notice the sensation of energy in the belly.

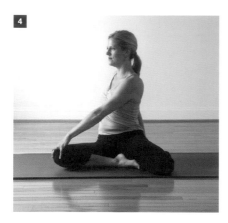

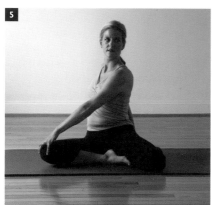

BHARADVAJASANA

This pose is a wonderful twist for all individuals, and is safe for any phase of the fertility cycle. It is also one of the only safe twists during pregnancy. Rishi means "divinely inspired sage" in Sanskrit and this twist helps us become aware of our innate wisdom and compassion.

1. Begin seated with legs outstretched in front of you. Sit on a blanket if it's difficult to keep a straight spine.

2. Bring the heel of your right foot into the groin, with the sole of the foot against the inner left thigh, and fold the left leg alongside the body. The top of the left foot should be tucked along the left hip, the sole of the left foot facing the ceiling.

3. With the heel of the right foot pressing firmly against the pelvic floor and both sitting bones fully grounded, sit tall. Move your attention down toward the floor through the perineum and sitting bones and then lift your ribcage away from your hip bones, gently pulling belly button to spine. The front knee can gently lift away from the floor in order to firmly ground the sitting bones.

4. Reach your right hand behind you to the floor. Inhale the left arm up by the ear and with an exhale take the left hand to the right knee.

5. Inhale again, making the spine long and tall and then exhale, twisting the torso and shoulders to the right and looking gently over the left shoulder. Do not torque or strain the neck here.

6. Take 10–20 breaths here, inhales making the spine long, exhales deepening the twist.

7. Gently release the pose and stretch the legs forward, bouncing them gently.

Repeat other side.

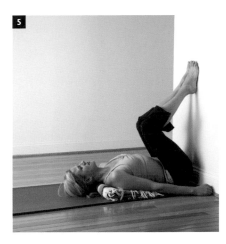

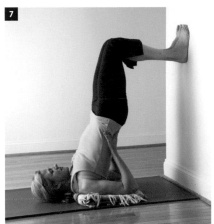

SALAMBA SARVANGASANA (SUPPORTED SHOULDER STAND)

We do not recommend practicing inversions during your menstrual period.

1. Lie on the floor with your legs up the wall, sitting bones as close to the wall as possible.
2. Take note of where your shoulders are on your mat and then come back to a seated position.
3. Place your folded blanket where your shoulders will be.
4. Now, lie down again with legs up the wall, sitting bones as close to the wall as possible. The blanket should support your shoulders and the back of the head should be on the floor. Play a bit until you get the support just right.
5. Slide your feet down until the soles of the feet are flat on the wall.
6. With an inhale, lift the hips, tuck the pelvis in, and press the soles of the feet into the wall. Gently roll the shoulders under and move the shoulder blades towards each other as you lift into Supported Shoulder Stand.
7. Walk the feet up the wall until the shins are parallel to the floor and bring the hands to support the lower back.
8. Breathe here, continuing to ground the shoulders down, scoop the tailbone, and bring the chest closer to the chin.
9. Hold for 20–30 breaths.

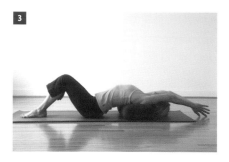

3

SUPPORTED MATSYASANA (FISH)

This counter-pose to Supported Shoulder Stand is wonderful for balancing the thyroid as well as opening the heart center to release sadness and anxiety. You will need a bolster or a rolled blanket to do this restorative pose.

1. Sit on your yoga mat with your knees bent, soles of your feet on the floor.
2. Lie back onto a bolster or rolled blanket so that the bolster is supporting your upper back and your head is free to stretch back and rest on the floor. If it feels uncomfortable to lie like this, or if the stretch feels too intense on your neck, place a towel under the head to lessen the bend in the neck.
3. Take your hands in front of the heart in prayer and then stretch them up over your head toward the floor.
4. Take 10–20 breaths.
5. To come out of the pose, bring your hands back to your heart and then release them on the floor. Gently scoot your shoulders off the bolster so your head is now resting on the support, as on a pillow.
6. Roll to your right side and rest here for a few breaths before returning to seated.

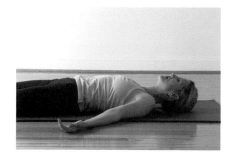

RELAXATION, OR SVASANA

Svasana is the final, and most important, pose of our yoga practice. In Svasana all the physical, energetic and emotional work of practice is processed and our bodies have time to rest and restore.

Mood Elevation

These postures, when done regularly, focus on opening your heart chakra, decreasing stress, and bringing positive energy into your body. Do this practice whenever you are feeling sluggish, down in the dumps, or unable to get out of bed.

Mood Elevating Practice

You can begin this practice on its own or, as time allows, start with 3 rounds of Moon Salutations.

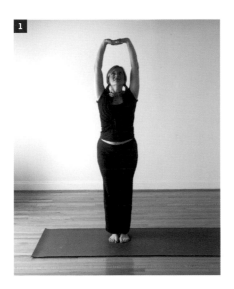

ARDHA CHANDRASANA

1. Inhale and lift your arms up over your head, turning the palms up to face the ceiling.
2. Stretch long, even lifting onto your tiptoes.
3. Grab your right wrist with your left hand. Exhale, take your hips to the right and your arms to the left. Hold for 5 breaths. In this posture you want to look like the crescent shaped moon shining in the evening sky.
4. Inhale and come back to center with your arms
5. Exhale and take your left wrist with your right hand. Lean to the right and stretch the left side of your body. Hold again for 5 breaths.
6. Come back to center.

Repeat this sequence 2 more times.

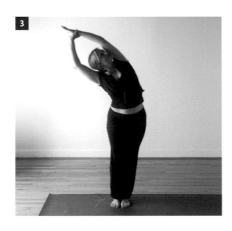

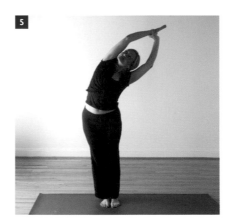

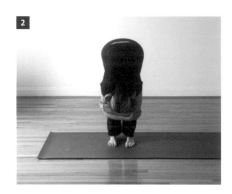

UTTANASANA

1. Place your feet hip-distance apart.
2. Hold opposite elbows and bow forward. Hold for 10 full breaths.

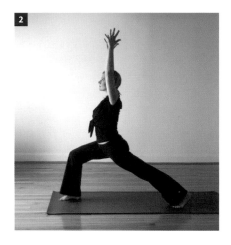

VIRABHADRASANA I VARIATION

1. Take your right foot forward and step your left leg back.
2. Bend your right knee so it aligns with the top of the right ankle. Come onto the ball mount of your left foot and raise your arms up alongside your ears. You can arch your back a bit and open your heart if it feels okay for your body. Hold for 5 breaths.

Repeat on the other side with the left foot forward and the right leg back.

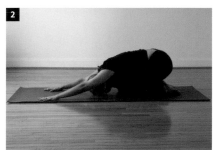

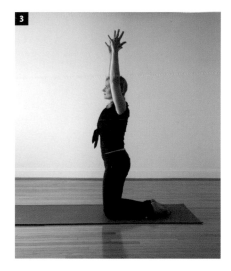

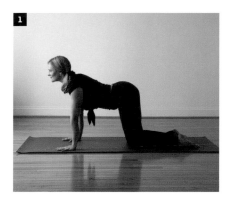

HAPPY CHILD SEQUENCE

1. Place your hands under your shoulders and your knees beneath your hips. Sink your chest without collapsing your shoulders. Arch your back slightly but keep the belly firm. Take an inhale in this posture, called "Table."
2. Exhale and move your stomach toward your thighs and your forehead to the ground in Child Pose (Balasana).
3. Inhale and lift your body off your legs and your arms upward alongside your ears.
4. Exhale back into Child Pose. Now you are back at step 1.

Repeat this sequence of four postures at least 5 times.

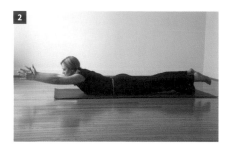

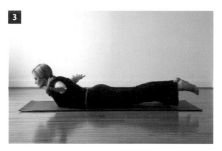

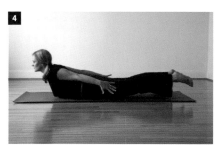

SALABASANA (LOCUST) SERIES

1. Lay on your belly (unless you are stimulating, bloated, or feel uncomfortable in doing so).
2. Inhale and lift your feet and hands off the ground by using the muscles in your abdomen and low back. Only your stomach will be on the ground with the legs touching at the thighs, knees, and ankles. Look straight ahead and allow the neck to be soft. Hold for 5 breaths and then release on an exhale.
3. Inhale again and lift up, keeping your arms and legs lifted. This time move your hands out to the side in a "T" position. Hold for 5 breaths and release on an exhale.
4. Finally, lift on an inhale and move your hands behind you so that they are alongside your body, keeping your legs lifted all the while.
5. Exhale and release your arms and legs. Now rest for a few breaths by making a pillow for your head with your hands.

Repeat this Salabasana sequence 3 times.

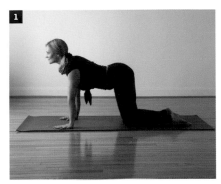

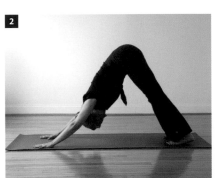

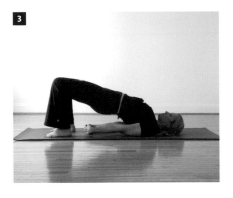

DOWNWARD FACING DOG

1. Place your hands on the mat, shoulders' width apart.
2. Exhale and bring your hips up toward the ceiling in an inverted "V" shape. Straighten the knees as much as your hamstrings permit and press your heels toward the mat. Hold for 5 breaths.

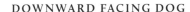

SETU BANDHASANA (BRIDGE)

1. Roll over onto your back and place your feet hip-distance apart and flat on your mat. Point the toes forward so that your feet are parallel to one another.
2. Inhale and lift your hips up toward the ceiling. Curl your shoulders toward each other on your back and, if your hands are available, clasp them together and use this leverage to move your hips and navel up higher toward the ceiling.
3. Hold for 10 inhales and exhales and then release.

Repeat 2 more times.

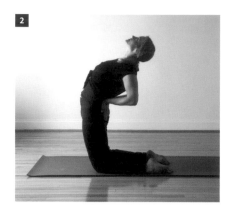

USTRASANA (CAMEL)

1. Kneel on the floor with the tops of your feet flat and toes pointing behind you. Keep the thighs together. Knees and feet can be comfortably separated.
2. Rest the palms on your hips, lift the ribs, exhale and then curve the spine backward toward your feet. Look up toward the ceiling if it feels safe for your neck. Hold for 3–5 breaths and then rest by simply sitting on your heels.

Repeat Camel 2 more times.

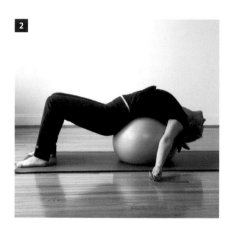

SUPPORTED BACKBEND

This pose is contra-indicated for those with neck pain or injury.

1. If you have a large exercise ball like the one pictured, sit on it and then gently roll it under your sacrum so that it supports your low back. Melt your spine onto the ball and let your head and neck release.
2. Take your arms out to the side and simply breathe, focusing on the sounds of your inhales and exhales. Stay as long as you like.

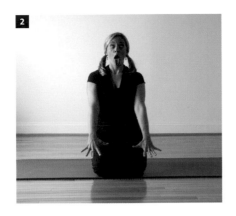

SIMHASANA (LION)

You might want to practice this one alone as you will you look quite funny doing it!

1. Sit on your heels with your spine nice and straight. Tighten the muscles of your face and stick your tongue out toward your chin as far as you can. Simultaneously, lift your brow and cross your eyes so that they are looking between your eyebrows or at the tip of your nose.
2. Stretch your arms out in front of you and open the fingers wide. Growl like a lion if you like. Hold the posture for a few breaths while breathing through the mouth.

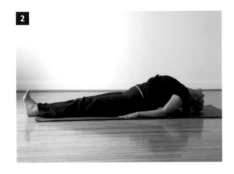

MATSYASANA (FISH)

1. Lie on the floor with your arms alongside you with a slight bend in your elbow.
2. On an exhale press your arms into the mat and arch the body back by lifting the chest and neck. Come onto the crown of your head and let it rest on the ground. Stay for 5 breaths.
3. To come out of the posture, push your forearms into the ground and lift your head first, thus allowing you room to straighten your back.

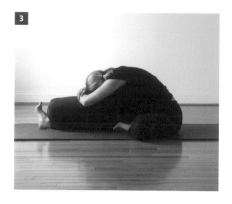

JANU SIRSASANA (HEAD TO KNEE POSE)

1. Sit down and extend your right leg forward.
2. Bend your left knee and take it out to the left side while bringing the sole of your left foot to the inner right thigh.
3. Exhale and bow forward by hinging at the waist and grabbing either the shin or ankle. For a more restorative posture, use a prop, like the bolster shown or a pillow, and rest your head on your prop. Hold the posture for 10 breaths.

Repeat on the other side by extending the left leg forward and bending the right knee.

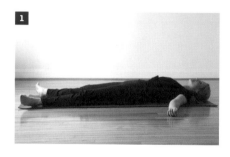

SAVASANA (CORPSE)

1. Lie on your back, letting the feet flop open and the arms to rest out to the side.
2. Dissolve into the earth and stay as long as you like.

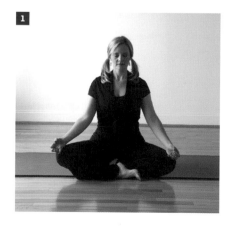

MEDITATION

1. After you have completed your savasana, sit quietly in a comfortable cross-legged seated position for at least five minutes.
2. State an intention or say a prayer to lock in the positive and enlivening energy you have just created through your practice.

THE CLEANSING POWER OF EXERCISE

For many women who come to Pulling Down the Moon, exercise has become a source of stress rather than a stress reliever. They may also be hearing conflicting messages from their doctor and at the gym on what's appropriate during infertility and IVF treatments. For this section, we worked with fertility doctors to come up with exercise guidelines that are both practical and safe during this time.

Tips for Fertility-Friendly Fitness

Emphasize low-impact, moderate-intensity cardiovascular exercise. Avoid sports that pound the body, such as running or high-impact aerobics, as these activities can create high levels of endorphins, the endogenous pain-killing chemicals that disrupt reproductive function. High intensity cycling, such as spinning, can also be highly intense, so hop on your bike for a leisurely spin through the forest preserve, swim a few laps in the pool, or go out for a walk instead.

RESISTANCE TRAINING

Perform resistance training with moderate weights. This will help maintain lean body mass, muscle tone, and bone health. There may be specific points during your medicated fertility cycle (like immediately post-transfer) where resistance training should be curtailed. Always follow your physician's instructions.

INCORPORATE YOGA INTO YOUR REGIMEN

Yoga helps with the detoxification process. The gentle stretches help release toxins from stagnant body tissues and can help promote elimination of toxins from the physical body.

REST AND RECOVERY

Take time for adequate time for rest and recovery. One of the first signs of "over-training syndrome" is an increase in levels of the stress hormone cortisol, a hormone that's not associated with optimal fertility! Cross-training—the practice of alternating the kinds of exercise you do every day—will allow for appropriate recovery if done wisely. Don't walk on the treadmill every single day: alternate with yoga and strength training to ensure that you are not overworking a particular muscle or group of muscles.

RELAXATION TRAINING

Stress is an inflammation-producing state. Training your body and mind to relax is a key component to any fertility-friendly fitness program. Practice meditation, conscious breathing, deep relaxation, and other activities that relax and refresh your body and mind.

To allay the worries of those of our patients using medical fertility treatment, we worked with our doctor partners to create the following guidelines for exercise during an ART cycle:

Pre-Stimulation
- Moderate physical activity is appropriate when preparing for A.R.T.
- Moderate exercise = 3-4 exercise sessions per week for 30-45 minutes per session.
- Recommended exercises: low-impact activities such as walking, swimming, yoga, biking, and strength training.
- Avoid impact activity such as running, jumping rope, cardio boxing, or impact aerobics.

During Stimulation
- Continue with mild physical activity (less intense sessions) as long as you are not experiencing discomfort or pain in the pelvic area.
- Lower the intensity of your workouts and avoid abdominal crunches and Pilates-type "core work" from the start of stimulation through the end of the cycle.
- If you are experiencing pelvic discomfort, STOP! If discomfort is severe or persists, always consult your physician.

Post-Retrieval
- Patients differ enormously in their experience of egg retrieval. Some experience a significant amount of discomfort and swelling; others experience little or no effects at all.
- Refrain from physical exercise for 48 hours post-retrieval to allow for any discomfort to subside.
- Wait until any swelling, discomfort, or inflammation dissipates before resuming even mild physical activity.

Post-Transfer
- Refrain from physical exercise for 48 hours post-transfer.
- After 48 hours, the resumption of gentle physical activity is permissible in the absence of pain, inflammation or other side-effects of treatment.
- Gentle, low-impact activity (walking, swimming, yoga) during the "two-week wait" period is appropriate.
- Physical activity will not impede embryo implantation or make an embryo "fall out."
- If any activity causes pain or discomfort, STOP!
- Avoid becoming short of breath, dehydrated or over-heated.
- Your pulse rate should be no more than 65% of estimate maximum heart rate pulse (usually 120 beats per minute is a good estimate).
- Avoid hot baths or Jacuzzis.

CHAPTER 11

The Cleansing Power
of the Breath

In simplest terms, the breath is the link between the body and mind and is the only body function under both conscious and unconscious control. When we bring our awareness to the breath, we break the spell of the automatic and unconscious. Deep, conscious breathing work, or pranayama, can reduce blood pressure and slow the pulse, reverse the physical symptoms of the Stress Response, and halt our association with negative thought patterns and mental habits.

Tips for creating and sustaining a regular breathing practice

- Take at least one week and do only the basic belly breathing. Practice mindfully, becoming aware of patterns of tension you might be holding in the body. Become comfortable with controlled and even breathing. Your yoga practice should help support this work.
- When you feel confident in your ability to consciously control deep breathing, move into the deeper breath practices. Use Resurrection Breath for new beginnings, Kapalabhati to create heat or when you are feeling sluggish, Sitali to help cool down, and Mental Alternate Nostril breathing to help you gain insight and clarity.

We have included a range of techniques that produce different physical and energetic effects. In this way, your breathing practices can become like a Chinese restaurant menu, where you mix and match according to your daily needs.

Basic Belly Breathing (To Relax)

Take a few minutes each day to focus on your breath and identify your breathing pattern. Try this exercise for deep, belly breathing:

STEP 1:   Sit in a straight-backed chair with your feet flat on the floor or lie down.
STEP 2:   Place one hand on your belly.
STEP 3:   Close your eyes and begin to breathe in and out through your nose.
STEP 4:   Breathe deeply into the abdomen, feeling your belly expand with the inhale.

STEP 5:   As you exhale, feel the hand and the belly gently move back toward the spine.

Continue this breathing pattern for 5-10 minutes. It may be helpful to visualize a balloon behind the navel that you inflate with the in-breath, and empty with the out-breath. With practice, this will become your habitual breathing pattern and you will reap the fertility benefits of relaxation, circulation, and a serene mind.

The Resurrection Breath (To Start Anew)

This quick and easy breathing sequence is meant to symbolically represent the death of one thing and the birth of another. The death could be your ego self, the death of a bad experience or the ending of something (like your day). The resurrection could be the rebirthing of a happier self, a better attitude, or new event.

To perform the technique, simply turn your head over your left shoulder and exhale quickly two times. This should empty all the air out of your lungs. In yoga, this is referred to as an empty chalice. Then, turn your head forward and inhale deeply, feeling the breath move down your spine and into your belly. As the breath fills your body again, it is referred to as full chalice. Continue long, slow belly breathing as long as you like after the Resurrection Breath ritual has been completed. Incorporate this ritualistic and purifying breathing practice before any breathing exercise, your yoga practice or even in the doctor's office before or after a consult.

THE DEEPER BREATHING PRACTICES

Cleansing Breath - Kapalabhati Pranayama - Breath of Fire (to Create Heat in the Body)

Kapalabhati is considered a cleansing and heat-generating breathing practice in yoga. It is believed to stoke the internal energetic fire (agni) inside and burn off negative energy, thoughts, or destructive patterns. It is also the best breath to do in the winter or when you feel cold or need additional warmth. Performing 25-30 cycles should heat you up nicely. Kapalabhati can also be used to create extra heat, so use it when you are feeling sluggish, tired, or feeling in need of a little "pick-me-up."

Here are step-by-step instructions. Come on, baby, light your fire!

STEP 1:   Sit comfortably on a chair or on the floor.
STEP 2:   Place your hand on your belly and see if you can exhale and simultaneously pull your hand and abdomen in toward your spine. At first you can exhale slowly and

focus your attention on drawing that belly inside. Then, after a bit of practice, begin to forcefully and quickly exhale with the abdomenal contractions at the same time. Notice how your belly contracts and pushes air out of your diaphragm and lungs. When you release the exhale and contraction, the body naturally breathes an inhale. As you become more adept at doing this practice, you will see how the breath and belly move together in symphony creating heat in the body. Those veteran Kapalabhati breathers can place their hands face up on their lap or knees, if they are familiar with the sensation of the belly moving out and in.

STEP 3:   Close your eyes, face forward, and tilt your chin down slightly.

STEP 4:   Take a Resurrection Breath before beginning your practice. Exhale quickly and frequently simultaneously pumping your belly to push air out of your lungs. Try exhaling 8-10 times in a 5-second interval. Naturally allow the body to inhale in between your controlled exhales. The inhales should happen naturally.

STEP 5:   Start slowly and work your way up to a 1-2 minute breathing practice. Remember: If at anytime you feel light-headed or dizzy, stop the practice and return to normal breathing. Next time, you will reduce the intensity or duration of your practice until any feelings of discomfort or dizziness dissipate.

Cooling Breath - Sitali Pranayama (To Cool Off)

This breathing practice does the exact opposite of Kapalabhati breathing. While Kapalabhati is referred to as the breath of fire, Sitali is considered the cooling breath. Sitali pranayama is meant to cool the sytem, reduce anxiety, and slow down the central nervous system. If you are feeling particularly frustrated or angry, sitali can help reduce this internal fire. Sitali is also helpful in reducing body heat during months of high seasonal outdoor temperatures and can be especially useful for women experiencing hot flashes or hormonal surges.

STEP 1:   Sit in a comfortable, relaxed position.

STEP 2:   Stick your tongue out and curl the sides upward so the tongue makes a tube.

STEP 3:   Hold the tongue in place with your teeth.

STEP 4:   Relax the lips as much as possible.

STEP 5:   Inhale long, slow deep breaths through the mouth so that the inhale passes through the tube you have made with your tongue. You should be able to feel the air hitting the tongue and passing through into the mouth.

STEP 6:   At the bottom of your inhale, retract the tongue back into the mouth and exhale slowly through the nose. During the exhale push the tongue far back into the mouth and up toward the roof so that the tongue gets moistened once again by your saliva.

STEP 7:   Stick your tongue out, make a tube shape, and inhale again through the mouth.

STEP 8:   Retract the tongue, moisten it, and exhale through the nose.

If you are doing sitali correctly, within four minutes time you should feel like someone just draped a large, cool, damp sheet over your entire body. See, there's a reason our canine friends stick their tongues out and pant when they get hot!

Mental Alternate Nostril Breathing (for Clarity)

This breathing technique is considered a cleansing breath and will help with mental balance. It is also good for unblocking minor sinus congestion in the nostrils. If you feel discomfort or light-headed when you are practicing, stop and return to your normal breathing pattern. No breathing technique should ever feel forced or uncomfortable.

STEP 1:   Sit comfortably with an erect spine and begin inhaling and exhaling through the nose.

STEP 2:   Imagine, with closed eyes, that as you inhale you are bringing in a blue stream of air into the right nostril only. As you exhale the blue stream of air exits the left nostril.

STEP 3:   Pause slightly at the completion of the exhale. Imagine inhaling the next breath through the left nostril and exit out the right. Pause. Inhale right, exhale left. Pause. Inhale left, exhale right.

STEP 4:   All of the breathing is done through the nostrils. The throat is not involved at all. Practice mental alternate nostril breathing for at least five minutes or as long as you like provided you feel calm and comfortable throughout the practice.

LIMBIC SYSTEM TRAINING

As you will recall from the first section of the book, the limbic system controls stress and relaxation in response to sensory input; therefore, we can use sensory input such as aromatherapy or music to train the nervous system to relax. Try introducing a sensory stimulus prior to one of your breathing practices for five minutes. Work your way through all the senses to see what might work best for you. With consistent practice, eventually just seeing, hearing, or touching this sensory input will stimulate relaxation at any time of day. Here are some examples for relaxing sensory stimuli for each of the five traditional senses:

SMELL: Using aromatherapy during relaxation sessions can create an association between relaxation and aroma. Calming scents include lavender, vanilla, ginger, and sandalwood.

HEARING: Listening to calming music, particularly music without lyrics in your language, can be deeply soothing.

SIGHT: Relaxing in a beautiful environment or gazing at a sunset can be deeply calming. Even lava lamps, with their beautiful colors and hypnotic movement, can promote peace.

TASTE: Try this wonderful meditation: See how long you can take to eat one raisin (or chocolate chip) while fully enjoying its texture, flavor, and smell. Take time to mindfully enjoy one taste prior to your relaxation session.

TOUCH: Self-massage is a wonderful way to send the "all-clear" signal to your brain. Here's a simple head massage that can stimulate clarity and relaxation. Let your fingertips meet at the midline of the skull, where the base of your skull (the occiput) meets your neck. Now, with gentle pressure massage the center line of the skull up and over the head toward the crown and finally the forehead.

CHAPTER 12

The Cleansing Power
of Awareness

Each of the following exercises, in their own way, creates Awareness. Sometimes the Awareness is that you have beliefs that cloud your perception of the world around you. Often, the Awareness is that you have habitual patterns that cause you to have repetitive negative outcomes over and over. And, in some cases, you have the Awareness that something exists inside you that is pure and divine. These exercises are meant to be meditations in some cases and rituals in others.

Exercise No. 1: Manifesting a Different Reality

Try the exercise below to see how the power of your thought forms might manifest your reality.

STEP 1:   Write down three negative things or characteristics you believe to be true about yourself. Please write these down before proceeding to step 2 or the exercise will not work.

STEP 2:   Ask yourself the following questions: Why do you think these characteristics are true and describe you accurately? Did someone do an experiment, or did you take a test that shows you are scientifically the characteristics you claim to be? Is this situation permanent? How do you know? Did someone tell you that you are these things and now you believe them? Did you decide for yourself that you are these things and now, therefore, you believe them?

STEP 3:   Do you really know for sure that you are the characteristics that you use to describe yourself?

STEP 4:   Are you 100 percent sure that these characteristics are really you?

STEP 5:   Ask yourself, "Who would I be if I did not believe these things were true about myself?"

STEP 6:   Could I be happier if I changed the negative perception of who I am?

STEP 7:   Could I be healthier if I changed the negative perception of who I am?

STEP 8:   Is it possible that I have created these negative beliefs about myself and, if I did, is it possible that the complete opposite might also be true?

Exercise No. 2: Planting Positive Thoughts

Channeling our power in the right direction is an important part of cleansing the mind. Often during the fertility process, we find our attention turns to incessant thoughts of struggle, hardship, frustration, or disappointment. It is important not to let the energy of these emotions draw in additional thoughts of powerlessness. In this exercise, you will be asked to do a visualization in which you plant seeds of positive intentions and then watch them grow before your mind's own eye.

STEP 1:   Find a comfortable seat and close your eyes.

STEP 2:   Focus for a few moments on the sound of your breath.

STEP 3:   Once the mind is settled, imagine you are walking amid vast farmland with dark, rich, nutritious soil stretching as far as the eye can see.

STEP 4:   Pick the soil up in your hand. Look at its richness, smell its aroma, feel its texture, slightly taste its pure earthiness.

STEP 5:   Release the soil in your hand. Now bend down and begin to dig out three holes in this rich soil, using only your hands as a digging implement.

STEP 6:   Speak a positive wish, desire, or prayer and drop the seeds of this intention into the first hole. Do the same for the remaining two holes.

STEP 7:   Cover all three holes with the soil.

STEP 8:   Watch the sky as a rain cloud passes above you and waters your seeds.

STEP 9:   See how the seeds begin to sprout and push up, out of the ground.

STEP 10: Notice how large your plants of intention are becoming. Feel them, smell them, taste them.

STEP 11: Stay in this moment as long as you like.

STEP 12: When you are ready, leave your plants to grow and flourish as you end your visualization.

Exercise No. 3: It's My Story, Damn It

Our wise friend and colleague, Dr. Marie Davidson, uses a technique in her own life and in counseling her fertility patients called "Narrative Psychology." She feels it's an effective way to help patients cope with the never-ending cycles of highs and lows that can accompany infertility. "At some point you realize that your life is your story," says Dr. Davidson. "It may not be the story you wanted to have, but it's yours and you have to stay in it. Sometimes the best you can do is simply watch the story unfold, but it's important to take ownership, be fully present, and feel confident it can have a happy ending."

Dr. Davidson asks her patients to spend a bit of time writing down what they thought life was going to be like, then write down what it is right now at this very moment. She then asks them to note the difference between what they imagined it would be and what it actually is. "Just because it might be different in some areas doesn't mean you don't still have a story; it's just that the story has changed," adds Dr. Davidson. "Note that in some areas the story might have turned out better than you imagined. Learn to embrace and take ownership of your story as it exists today."

Exercise No. 4: Finding Awareness

This exercise is meant to help you see if you can experience a little bit of that other part of yourself—the Awareness that is often clouded by our conscious minds.

1. Sit in a comfortable seated position either in a chair or on the floor with your back nice and straight.
2. Focus on an event or feeling that the conscious mind is currently struggling with. It could be your desire to have a child. It could be the project deadline your boss has given to you. Just think of an event that is currently challenging you.
3. What emotions do you feel as a result of this challenge? Acknowledge these emotions by either saying them to yourself or out loud.
4. When you think about one particular emotion, let's say it's anger, where do you feel it physically in your body? You may need to close your eyes to see if you can feel the anger somewhere in your physical self. This can be difficult because you are being asked to connect your mental thoughts with your physical body. Creating this bridge between the two will help you move farther down the rabbit hole of healing.
5. Focus on that part of the body that physically feels the emotion and think about what the opposite feels like. For instance, if you feel anger in your big toe, what would happiness feel like in your big toe? Remember: We all know the opposite of a feeling, so it is there inside you. Just concentrate on the physical sensation.
6. Now that you have brought the opposite feeling into your consciousness, can you remain in that feeling of happiness and step away from your big toe or that part of your body that was feeling the difficult emotion and look at it as an observer? When we say, "Step away," we are asking you to stay connected to the feeling of happiness, rather than continue to attach to your mind's thoughts or the physical sensations in the body.
7. After you have stepped away from the sensation can you say, "I am aware that right now the feeling of anger is present. I am observing the feeling of anger from a distance. I am a witness to anger."

When you become an observer or witness to your emotions rather than an active participant, you are connecting with Awareness. Again, Awareness is that part inside each of us that is pure, content, and in a constant state of peace.

Exercise No. 5: Becoming a Turtle

The ultimate goal in a mind cleanse is to figure out a way to transcend your toxic thoughts so you are able to use your mind as an organ of detoxification and tap into Awareness. This is not to say that we are trying to delete the negative experiences from our memory entirely; we are simply trying to neutralize them, look at them as an observer, and welcome the feelings and emotions they create in a nonreactive way. There is a Sanskrit term in yoga called pratyahara, which refers to being present but nonreactive. Since we now know that many of our experiences in life are created through our sensory perceptions, we can learn to withdraw from them in order to become a silent witness. Think of a turtle that pulls its legs and head inside of its shell. It closes itself off to all senses in order to be in the safety and tranquility of its own shell. This, in a sense, is pratyahara. An important distinction, however, is that the turtle must learn to transcend those sensory perceptions rather than withdraw from them or pretend they don't exist. Tami writes:

> *I regularly go to a yoga studio that is located adjacent to a canine grooming salon. Hearing those barking sounds during yoga has given my "down dog" a whole new meaning! At first, I was incredibly annoyed and wondered how anyone could have a peaceful or therapeutic yoga practice with all that commotion next door. It was a very annoying experience, particularly during savasana, when you are supposed to lie in corpse pose and turn off the world for those five luxurious minutes. I quickly realized that the agitation I was feeling and the resentment toward those darn barking dogs and the groomer was ruining my yoga experience. What if I stopped judging my experience because of those sounds and just accepted the fact that the dogs are going to bark? What a good exercise in pratyahara that would be, I thought. The barking dogs are not going away, so if I still want to do yoga in this lovely studio, I will have to learn to accept the fact that the dogs are going to bark. Now, when I hear those harsh sounds, I watch my reaction to the noise and then try to transcend the sound. I don't pretend the barking doesn't exist, I just choose not to react and be agitated any longer. It's funny, while I know the dogs are still barking, I really don't hear them anymore.*

Using Senses to Discover Awareness

Practice this exercise to heighten and experience the power of your senses. While it is best done in a busy location with a lot of action like an airport, train station or on a park bench, you can also practice this exercise right now, in the very room in which you are reading. The object is for you to see how your own senses contribute significantly to your view of the world.

1. What does this place look like? Experience everything with your eyes. What are the shapes, the colors, the designs and the patterns that you see. Drink up this place with the gift of your sight and turn your awareness solely to your eyes.

2. What does this place smell like? Close your eyes. Can you isolate different scents or sensations? Focus on your nose imagining the nostrils as tubular receptacles for the sense of smell. Do the smells remind you of something? Notice how your sense of smell can trigger memories from your past. Do not judge the memories or think too hard about what the smells might be. Just experience them.

3. What are the sounds that you hear? Open your ears fully and see if you can isolate the many noises surrounding you. Perhaps you can eavesdrop on a conversation or hear something in the background that was not otherwise apparent. What happens when you close your eyes? Can you hear better?

4. What do you feel with your hands in this location? Is the chair you are sitting upon soft or hard? Is the ground smooth or rough to the touch? Experience what you can through the sense of touch.

We trust by now you have had an opportunity to try the sensing exercise. What if we asked you to stop the sounds or the sights occurring in your location? You might laugh at us and say, "That's ridiculous; I can't stop 50 people from talking on a crowded bus nor could I make them vanish from my sight." You might be able to wear ear plugs or even repress the sound. You might be able to close your eyes and imagine they don't exist, but ultimately, you cannot get rid of the sound nor the sight. Similarly, we may be able to suppress various aspects of our selves such as emotions or a belief we hold to be true, but we cannot get rid of them.

It is much better to consciously allow everything to just exist as it is. Things are just the way they are anyway, right? This is an important tenent in learning to cleanse the mind. We must learn to accept things just as they are and life just as it is. When we accept and welcome all that is, conflict and challenges tend to go away because we don't put all that energy into fighting it. The restless mind becomes quiet and Awareness is experienced. Through this process of welcoming what is, we can begin to transcend our negative or toxic experiences and ultimately let go of those stories that no longer serve us.

Reliving the Past through Awareness

Whether we have been the target of abuse or have regretted our choices or actions from the past, there is a time in each of our lives when we wish we could turn back the hands of time and just fix it. A single event can become the foundation for a lot of angst, guilt and self-doubt. "If only I knew then what I know now," we might say, "I would press the rewind button, go into the past and make things right," or "I would have protected myself better from the person or action surrounding this event."

In the state of Awareness, time does not exist. It always was and always will be. In yoga, it is believed that if we can step into Awareness, we can call up a particular moment in time without bringing to the conscious mind the emotional baggage that comes along with it. Once you are able to enter this moment with detachment, you have the opportunity to neutralize the thoughts and emotions felt at that time. You relive it, so to speak, from the vantage point of your wisest self.

HOW IT WORKS

The concept is really quite simple. Let's say, for example, that you and your sister got into a horrible fight and you haven't spoken in years. You feel badly about it. Maybe you're not quite ready to reconcile, but you know that the emotions you feel from this event need to dissipate from your life. In this case, you would take the following steps:

1. Sit comfortably in a seated position.
2. Begin to breathe deeply, simply focusing on your inhale and exhale breaths.
3. When the mind begins to quiet and you feel ready, call to mind the troubling event. In this case, you are visualizing the moment you had the fight with your sister.
4. Imagine stepping into the conversation as your wisest self—loving, kind, but detached from emotion. Begin talking to your sister from Awareness and allow her to speak back to you. Listen to her side of the story. Send her love and blessings. Tell her why you acted the way you did, apologize, and mean it (even if it's not your fault). See if during this conversation she turns into Awareness, too.
5. Come out of the meditation and allow yourself to experience any feelings or emotions that are now present.

LET'S TRY ANOTHER EXAMPLE.

This time, let's say that someone physically hurt you. Call to mind the troubling event, conversation, or moment that just won't leave you. Through the process of visualization, imagine putting on a protective shield that covers the entire body. In the visualization, when the bees are coming near, the protective covering forbids them from injuring you. Visualize walking straight through a flurry of bees but not being affected by them. You feel strong, powerful, and fearless because of your protective covering.

The same technique can be used for all kinds of toxic memories. If you witnessed your cat getting run over, place a steel box around kitty and visualize the car rebounding off the box and moving away in the opposite direction. In your visualization, kitty's consciousness peacefully leaves the box uninjured and joyfully waves goodbye to you. We all know that kitty will not come back to us in physical form through this technique, but it may help you process and redirect the negative energy and toxic feelings you carry surrounding the event.

Bring into your meditation coats of armor, invisible shields, powerful weapons, magnetic forcefields, chastity belts, or anything else you might conjure up as a method of protection. While you may think this technique has its origins in a science fiction movie, we assure you that the meditation can be powerful in cleansing your memories.

We want to stress an important caveat: For some of you, the events that you experienced may be too painful to sit with for the purposes of this exercise. Please use common sense. If it has taken years of professional therapy to work through an event, it is advisable to keep working with your mental health care provider or discuss this technique with them prior to doing it.

THE CLEANSE LIFESTYLE CONTINUES

As we write this book, spring is once again and miraculously in full bloom after another long and challenging Chicago winter. Like life, like fertility, the cleanse lifestyle is ever evolving and changing. The areas of discussion in this book are the object of continuing research and debate in the medical and holistic communities. It is our intention to continue to develop methods, techniques and products that will help women walk a path of health, fertility and radiance. Be sure to visit our website from time to time as we post updates, videos, community events and relevant products that are meant to complement The Infertility Cleanse.

As always, you can share your experiences with us through our Facebook page or via "Contact Us" at *www.PullingDownTheMoon.com*.

We send you blessings on your journey.
Namaste,
Beth and Tami

REFERENCES CHAPTER 2

Angeli et al. (2004). "The overtraining syndrome in athletes: a stress-related disorder." Journal of Endocrinology Investigation, 27(6):603-12.

Bentov Y. et al. "The use of mitochondrial nutrients to improve the outcome of infertility treatment in older patients." Fertility & Sterility 2010;93:272–5.

Chavarro et al. (2007). "Diet and lifestyle in the prevention of ovulatory disorder infertility." Obstetrics and Gynecology. 110(5): 1050-8.

Chavarro et al. (2008). "Soy food and isoflavones intake in relation to semen quality parameters among men from a fertility clinic." Human Reproduction, 23(11):2584-90. Epub 2008 Jul 23.

Cordain et al. (2005). "Origins and evolution of the Western diet: Health implication for the 21st century." American Journal of Clinical Nutrition; 81: 341-354.

Doblado et al. (2007). "Glucose metabolism in pregnancy and embryogenesis." Current Opinion in Endocrinology, Diabetes and Obesity. 14(6): 488-493.

Evans, K. E. et al. (2009). "Be vigilant for patients with coeliac disease." Practitioner, 253(1722):19-22, 2.

Fernandez-Real JM et al. (1999) "Plasma oestrone-fatty acid ester levels are correlated with body mass in humans." Clinical Endocrinology. Feb;50(2):253-60.

Fraczek M et al. (2007). "Inflammatory mediators exert toxic effects of oxidative stress on human spermatozoa." Journal of Andrology, 28(2): 325-333.

Friebe A. et al. (2008). "Causes for spontaneous abortion: What the bugs 'gut' to do with it?" The International Journal of Biochemistry & Cell Biology, 40 : 2348–2352.

Gesink Law et al. (2007). "Obesity and time to pregnancy." Human Reproduction, 22(2): 414–420.

Hauser et al. (2008). "Urinary phthalate metabolites and semen quality: A review of a potential biomarker of susceptibility." International Journal of Andrology, 31(2):112-117. Epub 2007 Dec 6.

Laitinen et al. "Probiotics and dietary counselling contribute to glucose regulation during and after pregnancy: a randomised controlled trial." British Journal of Nutrition. 101, 1679-1687.

Levin et al. (2007). "Higher C-reactive protein levels during IVF stimulation are associated with ART failure." Journal of Reproductive Immunology. 75(2):141-144. Epub 2007.

REFERENCES CHAPTER 3

Bari et al. (2011). "The manifold actions of endocannabinoids on female and male reproductive events." Frontiers in Bioscience,16:498-516.

Cassidy A. et al. (1994) "Biological effects of a diet of soy protein rich in isoflavones on the menstrual cycle of premenopausal women." American Journal of Clinical Nutrition. 60:333-340.

Chavarro et al. (2009). Caffeinated and alcoholic beverage intake in relation to ovulatory disorder infertility. Epidemiology. 20, 374-81.

Chavarro et al. (2008). "Soy food and isoflavone intake in relation to semen quality parameters among men from an infertility clinic." Human Reproduction. 23(11):2584-2590.

Chen et al. (2009). "Regulation of energy metabolism pathways by and estrogenic chemicals and potential implications in obesity associated with increased exposure to endocrine disruptors." Biochimica et Biophysica Acta. 1793 (7):1128-1143.

Dolinoy et al. (2007) "Maternal nutrient supplementation conteracts bisphenol A-induced DNA hypo-methylation in early development." Proceedings of the National Academies of Science USA. 104 (32) 13056-61.

Eustache et al. (2009). Environ Health Perspect.,117(8):1272-1279. Epub 2009.

Foster et al. (2008). "Environmental contaminants and human infertility: Hypothesis or cause for concern?" Journal of Toxicology and Environmental Health Part B Crit Rev.,11(3-4): 162-176.

Ganmaa, D. et al. (2005). "The possible role of female sex hormones in milk from pregnant cows in the development of breast, ovarian and corpus uteri cancers." Medical Hypotheses 65, 1028-37.

Grant et al. (1991). Detoxification pathways in the liver. Journal of Inherited Metabolic Disease, 14 (4): 421-430.

Hauser et al. (2008). "Science linking environmental contaminant exposures with fertility and reproductive health impacts in the adult male." Fertility & Sterility. 89:59–65.

Kinney et al. (2007). "Smoking, alcohol and caffeine in relation to ovarian age during the reproductive years." Human Reproduction. 22(4):1175-1185. Epub 2007 Jan 29.

Lu LJ et al. (2001) "Effects of an isoflavone-free soy diet on ovarian hormones in premenopausal women." Journal of Clinical Endocrinology and Metabolism. 86, 3045-52.

Lu LJ et al. (1996) "Effects of soya consumption for one month on steroid hormones in premenopausal women: implications for breast cancer risk reduction." Cancer Epidemiological Biomarkers. 1, 63-70.

Mendola et al. (2008). "Science linking environmental contaminant exposures with fertility and reproductive health impacts in adult females." Fertility & Sterility. 89:81–94.

Parveen et al. (2010). Genetic association of phase I and phase II detoxification genes with recurrent miscarriages among North Indian women. Molecular Human Reproduction. 16(3):207-214.

Rossi et al. (2011). "Effect of alcohol consumption on in vitro fertilization." Obstetrics & Gynecology, 117(1), 136-142.

Spiroux de Vendomois, J et at. (2010). "Debate on GMOs Health Risks after Statistical Findings in Regulatory Tests." International Journal of Biological Sciences. 6(6):590-598.

Taioli et al. (2010). "Comparison of estrogens and estrogen metabolites in human breast tissue and urine." Reproductive Biology & Endocrinology. 8: 93.

Unfer et al. (2004). "Phytoestrogens may improve the pregnancy rate in in vitro fertilization–embryo transfer cycles: A prospective, controlled, randomized trial." Fertility and Sterility, 82(6): 1509-1513.

Whitcomb et al. (2010). Ovarian function and cigarette smoking. Paediatric Perinatal Epidemiology. 24(5):433-440.

Windham et al. (2005) "Exposure to organochlorine compounds and effects on ovarian function." Epidemiology. 16(2):182-90.

Xia et al. (2009). "Relation between urinary metabolites of polycyclic aromatic hydrocarbons and human semen quality." Environmental Science & Technology, 43(12):4567-4573.

REFERENCES CHAPTER 4

Fisher-Wellman et al. (2009). "Acute exercise and oxidative stress: a 30 year history." Dynamic Medicine, 8:1.

Klecolt-Glaser JK et al. (2010). "Stress, inflammation and yoga practice." Psychosomatic Medicine. 72(2):113-21.

Pitman R et al. (2002). "Pilot Study of Secondary Prevention of Post Traumatic Stress Disorder with Propranolol." Biological Psychiatry. 2002;51:189 –142

Ruder et al. (2008). "Oxidative stress and antioxidants: Exposure and impact on female fertility." Human Reproduction Update. 14(4): 345–357.

Shahin et al.(2008). "Adding phytoestrogens to clomiphene induction in unexplained infertility patients—a randomized trial." Reproductive Biomedicine Online. 16(4):580-588.

Sowers et al. (2006). "Selected Diet and Lifestyle Factors Are Associated with Estrogen Metabolites in a Multiracial/Ethnic Population of Women." Journal of Nutrition. 136:1588-1595.

Swithers et al. (2008). "A role for sweet taste: Calorie predictive relations in energy regulation by rats." Behavioral Neuroscience. 122(1): 161-173.

Veleva et al. (2008). "High and low BMI increase the risk of miscarriage after IVF/ICSI and FET." Human Reproduction, 23 (4), 878–884.

Verdu et al. (2009). "Between celiac disease and irritable bowel syndrome: The "no man's land" of gluten sensitivity." American Journal of Gastroenterology, 104(6):1587-1594.

Verstraelen, H. et al. (2005). Vaginal lactobacilli, probiotics, and IVF. Reproductive BioMedicine. 11 (6): 674–675.

Wakefield et al. (2008). "Maternal supply of omega-3 polyunsaturated fatty acids alter mechanisms involved in oocyte and early embryo development in the mouse." American Journal of Physiology and Endocrinology Metabolism. 294: E425–E434.

Wathes et al. (2007). "Polyunsaturated fatty acids in male and female reproduction." Biology of Reproduction. 77: 190-201.

Wu et al. (2004). "Glutathione Metabolism and Its Implications for Health." Journal of Nutrition. 134:489-492.

REFERENCES CHAPTER 5

Dalai Lama and Howard Cutler. The Art of Happiness (Riverhead, 1998).

Richard J. Davidson, PhD, Jon Kabat-Zinn, PhD, Jessica Schumacher, MS, Melissa Rosenkranz, BA, Daniel Muller, MD, PhD, Saki F. Santorelli, EdD, Ferris Urbanowski, MA, Anne Harrington, PhD, Katherine Bonus, MA and John F. Sheridan, PhD. Alterations in Brain and Immune Function Produced by Mindfulness Meditation. Psychosomatic Medicine. 65:564-570 (2003)

Friedmann, Erika, PhD, Sue A. Thomas, RN, PhD, FAANa, Fang Liu, MSa, Patricia G. Morton, RN, PhD, CANP, FAANa, Deborah Chapa, RN, MS, CRNPa, Stephen S. Gottlieb, MD, FACCc. (2006). The Relationship of Depression, Anxiety, and Social Isolation to Chronic Heart Failure Outpatient Mortality. American Heart Journal. 2006;152(5):940.e1-940.e8.

Fredrickson, B.L., Cohn, M.A., Coffey, K.A., Pek, J., & Finkel, S.M. (2008). Open hearts build lives: Positive emotions, induced through loving-kindness meditation, build consequential personal resources. Journal of Personality and Social Psychology. 2008, Vol 95, No 5, 1045-1062.

REFERENCES CHAPTER 7

Boivin, J. et al. (2011). Emotional distress in infertile women and failure of assisted reproductive technologies: meta-analysis of prospective psychosocial studies, British Medical Journal. Feb 23, 2011; 342:d223. doi: 10.1136/bmj.d223)

Imeson M and A. McMurray. (1996). "Couples' experiences of infertility: a phenomenological study." School of Nursing, Edith Cowan University, Churchlands, Perth, Western Australia. (1996) J Adv Nurs. Nov 1996; 24(5):1014-22.

REFERENCES CHAPTER 8

Adlerkreutz, H.(2007). "Lignins and human health." Critical Reviews in Clinical Laboratory Science. 44(5-6): 483-525.

Gleicher et al. (2010). "Miscarriage rates after dehydroepiandrosterone (DHEA) supplementation in women with diminished ovarian reserve: a case control study." Reproductive Biology & Endocrinology. 2010; 8:140.

Hollis et al. (2004). "Assessment of dietary vitamin D requirements during pregnancy and lactation." American Journal of Clinical Nutrition. 79:717–26.

Ozkan et al. (2010). "Replete vitamin D stores predict reproductive success following in vitro fertilization." Fertility & Sterility. 2010 Sep; 94(4):1314-9.

Papaleo et al. (2009). "Contribution of myo-inositol to reproduction." European Journal of Obstetrics & Gynecology and Reproductive Biology. 147: 120–123.

Papaleo et al. (2009). "Myo-inositol may improve oocyte quality in intracytoplasmic sperm injection cycles. A prospective, controlled, randomized trial." Fertility & Sterility. 91(5):1750-4.

Wiser et al. (2010). "Addition of dehydroepiandrosterone (DHEA) for poor-responder patients before and during IVF treatment improves the pregnancy rate: a randomized prospective study." Human Reproduction. 25(10):2496-500.

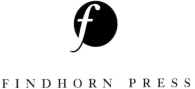

FINDHORN PRESS

Life Changing Books

For a complete catalogue,
please contact:

Findhorn Press Ltd
117-121 High Street,
Forres IV36 1AB,
Scotland, UK

t +44 (0)1309 690582
f +44 (0)131 777 2711
e info@findhornpress.com

or consult our catalogue online
(with secure order facility) on
www.findhornpress.com

For information on the Findhorn Foundation:
www.findhorn.org

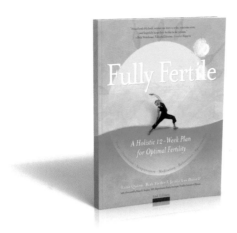

Fully Fertile 2nd Ed

A Holistic 12–Week Plan
for Optimal Fertility

The healing powers of traditional yoga, Oriental medicine, nutrition, and other mind/body techniques are accessible with this do-it-yourself manual for women who are struggling with infertility or just looking to improve their odds of conception. Natural methods based on Integrative Care for Fertility™ use a holistic approach to demonstrate how a home-based holistic fertility program can improve mind, body, and spirit, and in turn maximize chances for conceiving.

Photographs are provided to illustrate the proper yoga postures, and interspersed stories from yoga practitioners and experts present real-life struggles of infertility patients and victories that will inspire all women who are trying for a healthy pregnancy and birth. Includes a 16-page Fully Fertile Book Group Study Guide.

*Available at **www.findhornpress.com***
*or the authors' website, **www.pullingdownthemoon**.*
$19.95 · £12.99
ISBN 978-1-84409-507-0

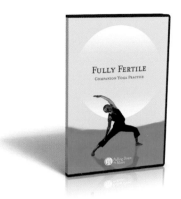

Fully Fertile DVD

Companion Yoga Practice

Breathe, stretch and cultivate a fertile lifestyle with this DVD which has been created as a companion to the books *Fully Fertile* and *The Infertility Cleanse*. There are seven easy-to-follow yoga sections that you can "mix and match" to create a practice that is customized to your needs. Taught by Pulling Down the Moon co-founders, Tami Quinn and Beth Heller, this DVD is easy to follow and requires no prior yoga experience.

For best results, we recommend that you practice yoga a minimum of 5 times per week for approximately 30-45 minutes at a time. You can combine any of the yoga segments on the DVD, but as a general rule each practice should start with Moon Salutes and end with resting pose. Here are several of our favorite practices:

Aid Digestion and Elimination
Moon Salutes + Samana Practice

**Improve Blood Flow
and Release Anxiety**
Moon Salutes + Apana Practice

**Manage the Blues
and Cultivate Positive Energy**
Moon Salutes + Mood Elevating Practice

Create Deep Relaxation
Breathing + Restorative Practice

*The DVD and other exclusive fertility-specific products can be purchased through our on-line boutique at **pullingdownthemoon.com***

In many ways this book is a call to become a pioneer, to begin to look at different ways we consume and create things. While our patterns of consumption and creation may or may be not be related to our ability to conceive, they are ultimately related to our ability to flourish. The ability to thrive is the ultimate definition of fertility.

That is what we mean by an Infertility Cleanse.